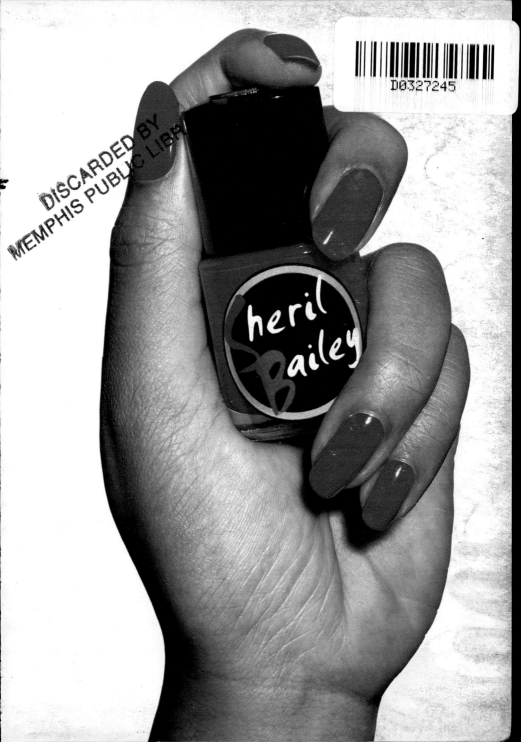

D0327245

Sheril
Bailey

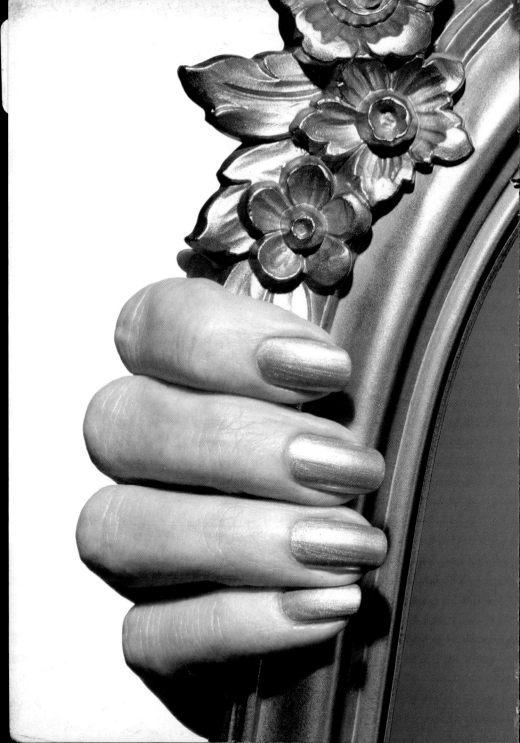

The *Sheril Bailey*
Complete Manicuring and Nail Care Handbook

written by
Sheril Bailey

photography by
Michael Thompson

creative direction and illustrations by
Donald F. Reuter

Andrews McMeel
Publishing
Kansas City

The Sheril Bailey Complete Manicuring and Nail Care Handbook
Copyright © 1998 by Sheril Bailey.

Produced by Alias Books.

Printed in Singapore.

Andrews McMeel Publishing
an Andrews McMeel Universal company
4520 Main Street
Kansas City, Missouri 64111

www.andrewsmcmeel.com

Library of Congress Cataloging-in-Publication Data

Bailey, Sheril.
        The Sheril Bailey complete manicuring and nail care handbook / written by Sheril Bailey ; photography by Michael Thompson ; creative direction and illustrations by Donald F. Reuter.
            p.   cm.
ISBN 0-8362-5187-3 (hardcover)
1. Nails (Anatomy)–Care and hygiene.   I. Title.
RL94.B35   1998
646.7'27–dc21

97-41545
CIP

Frontispiece: Classic red nails. Title page: Classic gold metallic nails. Opposite: A "manicuring bar" set up for female factory workers in London, England, during World War II. (photo courtesy of Hulton-Deutsch Collection/Corbis)

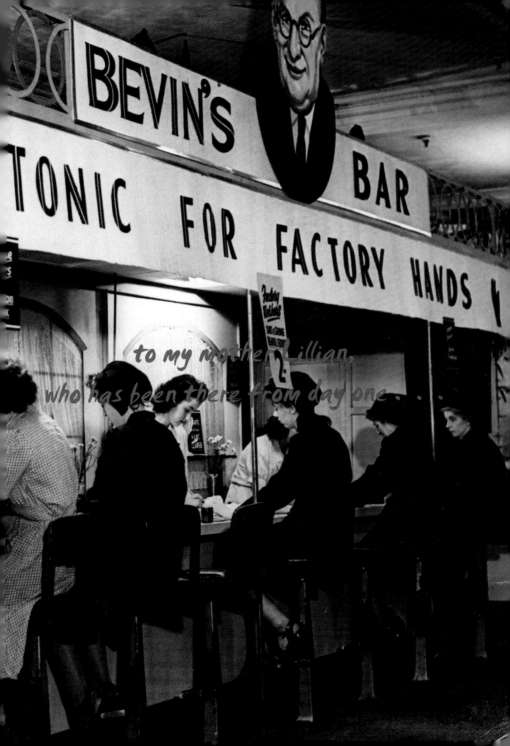

BEVIN'S BAR

TONIC FOR FACTORY HANDS

to my mother Lillian,

who has been there from day one . . .

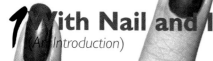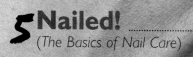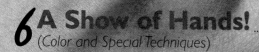

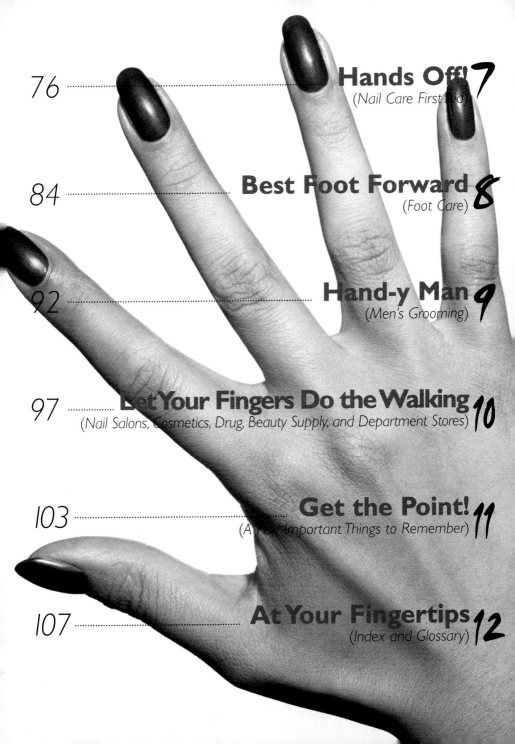

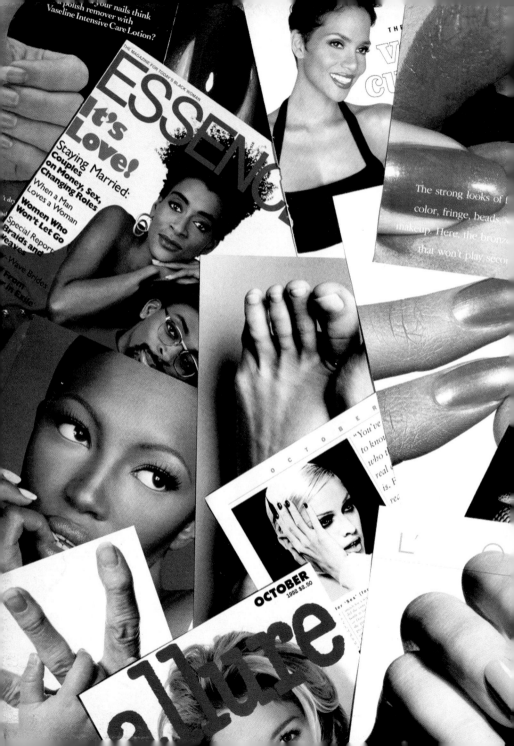

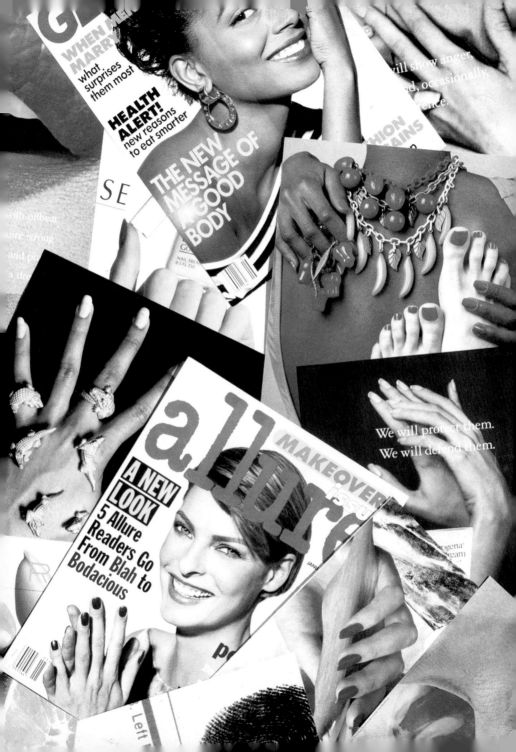

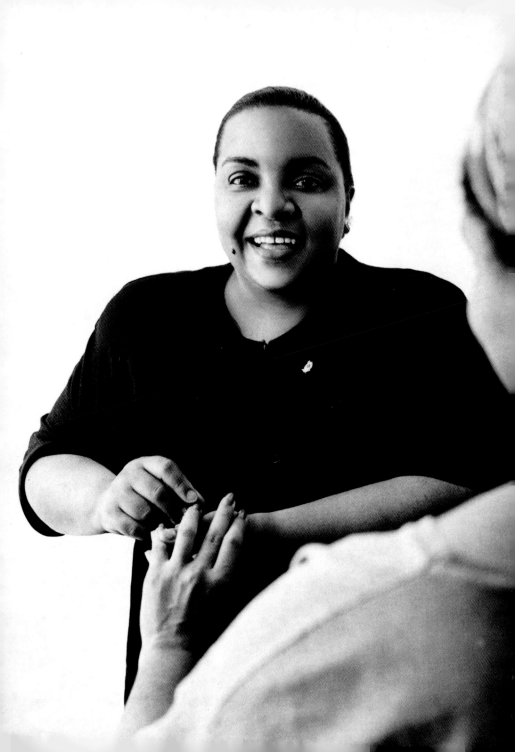

1 With Nail and I
(An Introduction)

Many people expect me, as a Jamaican-born woman with a bit of an island accent, to have a past brimming with tales of tropical lore. Unfortunately, by those standards, my life story turns out to be quite "normal." In my past there were no boats washing ashore, no political upheavals in the populace, and no vignettes of immigrant aggression. In fact, my life in Barbican Heights, Jamaica, was much the same as any young girl's around the globe. On my walls were photos of the Beatles and Toots and the Maytals; most of my dresses came from shopping trips my mother took to Miami. And, as with many a youngster, I didn't always know what I wanted to do. As I grew a bit older, I became more and more interested in the beauty business. At the time, my sister was living in Toronto, Canada, and was working her way up in civil engineering. I went to stay with her as a home base for my education in beauty. (I had planned to take these skills back to Jamaica, but my initial few years rapidly turned out to be a lifetime of great work.)

With my mother in tow as chaperone, I moved on to New York City. It was the early seventies and the sportswear fashion scene was about to blossom. The attention was shifting away from Paris as the center of the universe of style; designers like Halston, Calvin Klein, and Ralph Lauren were on their way to becoming household names. Manicures at that time were still thought of as a luxury, performed on only the richest and

Previous spread: A "collage" of some of my work highlights.
Opposite: That's me on the set with hand model Magdelene.

11

most important of female clientele and only in full-service salons in the company of some great coiffeurs. Intent on my career in the beauty business, I enrolled at Clara Barton's, a vocational high school in Brooklyn that specialized in beauty training. Originally, I had hoped to become a hairdresser, but I soon realized my talents were put to better use as a manicurist. My manner worked well with the customer, and it was not unheard of for me to sit with someone for an hour or so. (Remember, this was right before the advent of the working woman and her harried schedule.) I worked long hours, between salons and shoots, and my reputation grew. With each job, I gained the skills, techniques, and confidence that I would carry with me throughout the rest of my career.

Now, as a nail care specialist for many years, I have been fortunate (and proud) to have worked with some of the very best people in this business, from the hottest new models to the coolest celebrities, the hippest magazines to the most genius photographers, not to mention brilliant hairstylists and makeup artists. We all work in unison to create the beauty images that form the foundation of our industry. It is a very gratifying and exciting profession, filled with imagination and inspiration. To this day, I am still in awe when I see my work on a billboard, photo spread, or television screen. But I have also seen a lot come and go (and come again). Fashion and beauty is a spinning wheel that at times seems to change solely for the sake of change. It is because of this volatility that I have tried to remain constant and consistent and have, over the years, developed a signature "look" that I adapt accordingly to daily needs.

I often feel that nail care and manicuring are given short shrift where our fashion and beauty interests are concerned. While you will hear countless stories about a celebrity's dress at an award show, her new

One of my favorite "still life" photos. Here the nails are polished in a neutral tawny color and their shape is a classic oval.

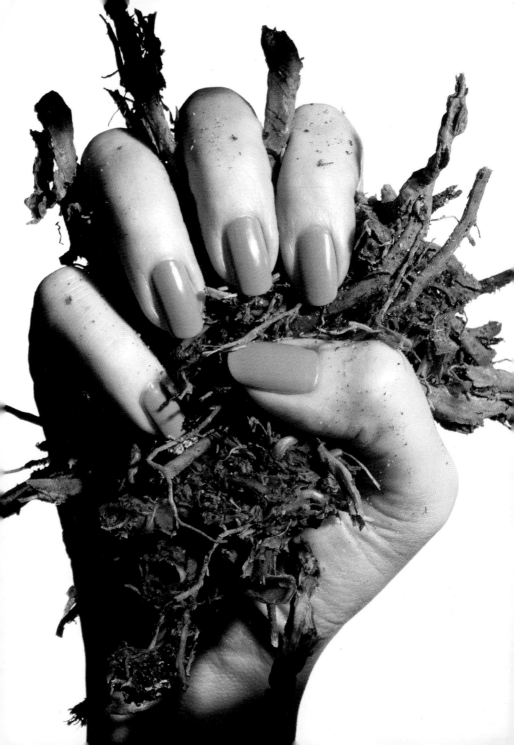

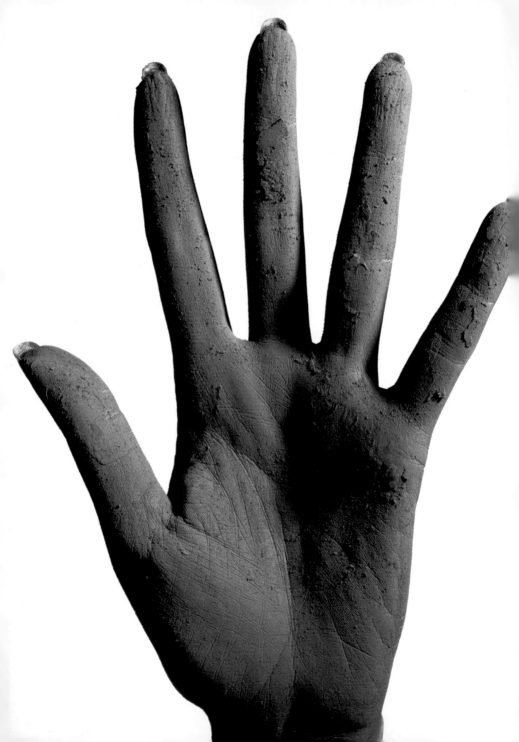

hairstyle or revamped face (cosmetically or surgically), you never hear a peep about her hands. Don't get me wrong. A manicure will never be especially newsworthy, except sometimes in the case of a star like Madonna, and I am not saying it should be. In fact, that would be rather silly. Personally, I like the fact that of all these different components—hair, makeup, outfit, and nails—your hands maintain the quietest profile, despite the fact that they must function and perform effortlessly. But, since these other areas visually dominate, your nails easily fall victim to neglect (or misguided attention, such as when they are grown to a ridiculously impractical length). In this book, I hope to remedy that problem. Follow my advice and, regardless of where or how you groom them, your nails will perform their many functions with grace and style while remaining care- and worry-free.

I think it's best to start with a basic understanding of good grooming and nail care. The techniques I have learned and practiced over the years are effective, yet uncomplicated. The most successful manicures, I find, are the ones with steps that are easy and simple. (If it looks difficult and fussy, it was probably difficult and fussy to do.) Now, with nail salons as abundant as fast-food restaurants, we have a whole new set of options open to us. The choices are limitless.

But remember, we're only talking about nails here, just one small physical part of the entire package that makes up who we are. It's important to keep a healthy perspective on these things, especially concerning beauty ideals. Sometimes, it can lose all sense of reality. I like to seek refuge in my family. With husband, mother, and two teenage children, I have plenty to keep me busy outside of "fashion." But, admittedly, even my daughter and her friends find a little enchantment in a simple glitter nail polish. And so do I.

Here, even though the nails only show from the back and the focus is on the dusting of blue pigment, the shape of the nail's free edge was of utmost importance—another favorite photo.

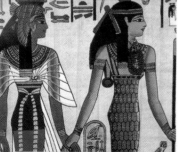

2 The Hands of Time

(A Brief Look Back at Nails)

The citizens of ancient Egypt and Babylonia were known to have "painted" their nails red and black. This included everyone from royalty, like Cleopatra, to male soldiers.

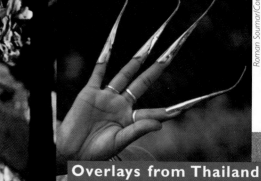

Overlays from Thailand that are still used today.

The Chinese are credited with the first known "polishes," although they were said to be more like paint. They also embellished and elongated the fingertips with gold overlays.

The word manicure comes from the Latin for hand (*mani*) and groom (*cura*).

The begloved hands and arms of the aristocracy.

Corbis-Bettmann

The unadorned but well-manicured hands of the courtesan and the novitiate.

Nails of the royal courts of England; always well groomed and buffed.

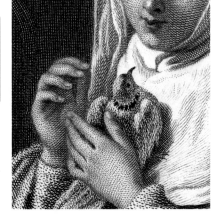

Back in the late 1800s, nails were groomed with a powdery substance that was buffed onto the nail in a polishing action. Hence the term nail "polish." Even though liquid-based products were introduced in the 1920s, the name has stayed with us.

Corbis-Bettmann

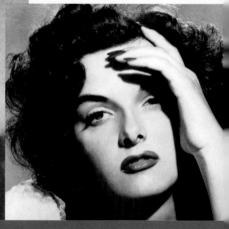

The "pinup" and her ubiquitous red nails.

With the popularity of liquid "polishes," new techniques of application were soon to follow, like these bicolored '30s nails.

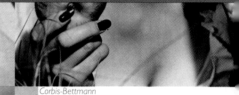

The unadulterated but luxuriously manicured hands of the sophisticated.

In many foreign countries the word varnish is used instead of **polish**.

The "go-go" sixties and bubble-gum pink . . .

The glamour girl of the fifties and her version of the lacquered nail.

. . . to the "disco-fied" seventies and glitter nails.

With the 1980s and the "punk" black nail, manicuring and nail care entered into a new era. By the ′90s, the popularity of at-home computers, nail salons, and quality products at affordable prices would see the "world" of nails moving easily into the twenty-first century.

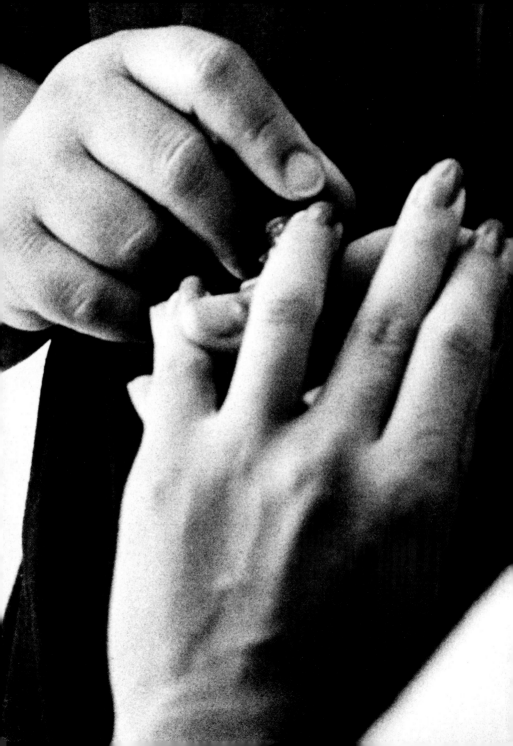

3 . . . Like the Back of Your Hand

(Simple Anatomy of the Nail)

I am not an anatomist, but I do know that a basic understanding of the fundamental structure and function of the nails (both hand and foot) can help with the development of the proper habits in their care and grooming. Moreover, good care and grooming habits keep nails in optimum working condition, which itself helps avoid problems down the road.

The nails are composed mainly of an organic substance called keratin. (Your hair is made up of the same matter.) Once keratin reaches the outside surface of the body, the cells are already dead. (*The very reason it doesn't hurt when you cut them!*) First and foremost, the nails are meant to **protect** the areas where they appear. And that's one *very* good reason why it is so important to maintain them in the utmost condition. Think of them as little shields that keep the tips of your fingers and toes from harm.

Internally, the structure of the hands (and feet) consists of these main parts: the skeleton, over which lie the muscles, and

A "close-up" detail from the photo on page ten.

the dermis and the epidermis, both of which contain nerves, nerve endings, and blood vessels. The hand itself is a relatively simple arrangement of twenty-seven bones leading from the wrist to the fingertips. (The feet contain twenty-six.) Each bone is connected to the next by a series of ligaments and muscles and cushioned by a small bit of cartilage. As we get older, wear and tear can cause hands and feet to become less flexible. (*Frequent massaging can help to lessen the impact of age. There are also some great exercises you can do on a regular basis to strengthen the small muscles.*) The hands in particular should be kept warm and moisturized, especially during the winter months, as colder air can limit circulation and dry out the skin. (The feet, however, should be kept warm, but dry.) Furthermore, use of moisturizers helps keep the skin soft and supple. This will also help prevent or minimize signs of aging, such as wrinkles and spotting.

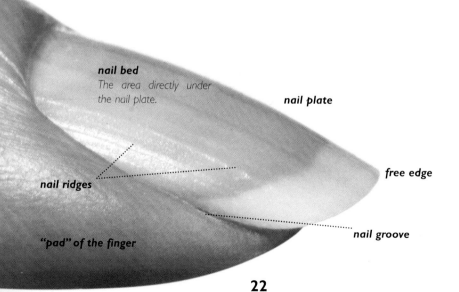

nail bed
The area directly under the nail plate.

nail plate

nail ridges

free edge

"pad" of the finger

nail groove

nail groove
The crease of skin through which the nail travels.

nail ridge
This clearly illustrates how a ridge will reflect the light differently than does the rest of the nail plate.

nail plate
The visible part of the nail.

free edge
The end of the nail, usually overhanging the fingertip.

cuticle
The piece of skin that overlaps the nail plate. Possible function: as a protection for the nail root and matrix.

nail root
The true base of the nail, originating at the matrix.

lunula
The whitish, crescent-shaped area, barely visible in this photo, is directly over the matrix. The coloring is due to light reflection.

nail mantle
The skin of the finger that protects the nail root.

nail matrix
The area that manufactures the nail. It contains nerves and blood vessels and is partially visible under the lunula. If you injure yourself here, it will likely show up as discoloration on the nail plate.

The hands are extraordinarily versatile tools; they should never be taken for granted.

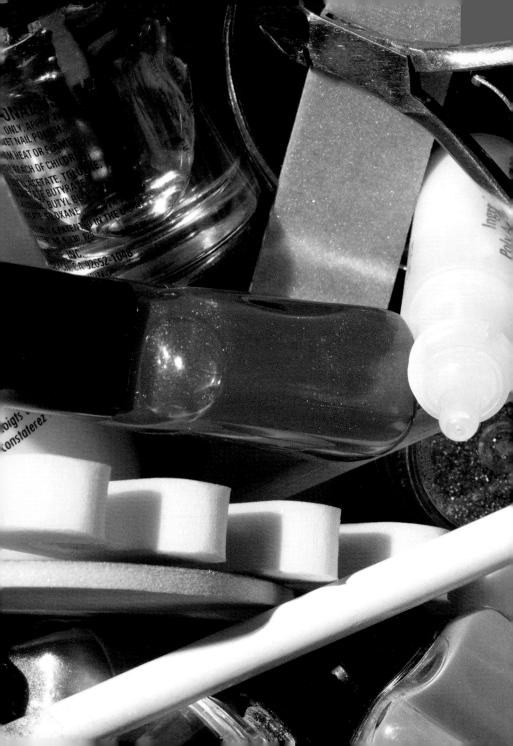

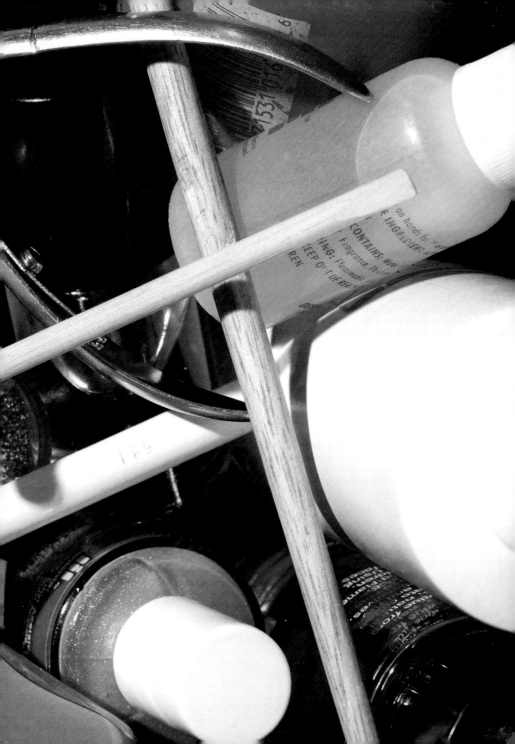

4 Keep It Hand-y!
(Tools and Products)

tools

Our hands are expected to perform innumerable tasks. However, it is possible to maintain them with a few carefully chosen implements and products. Over the years I have tried countless tools, polishes, and cremes. Many have fallen by the wayside, others I find I cannot do without. When choosing these things for oneself, I feel it is always best to go with what is most comfortable. Instruments, especially, should fit easily in the hand and around the fingers in order to perform smoothly. You may find that you can get along quite easily with just a few items, or you may have some additions of your own. Regardless of what you use, always replace tools when they have lost their efficiency. Remember, a pair of dull scissors and overused buffers can split, tear, and dry out your nails and do much more harm than good.

For my own professional and personal use, I find the following tools to be absolutely essential if I expect to create the perfect nail:

pumice stones (man-made)

nail scissors

emery boards

disk files

polish remover pads

(natural) cotton

white pencil

orangewood stick (and plastic version)

nail buffer (stick version)

nail stone (natural)

toe separator

cuticle nippers

magnifying glass

nail clippers (two versions)

toenail scissors

nail brush

nail buffer (handheld)

*(All items shown on the next few pages are slightly **smaller** than actual size.)*

pumice stones (man-made) - Both versions are for removal of excess skin, especially around the foot. The long-handled style allows for more freedom of movement, while the block style is more long-lasting. (Always rinse thoroughly after use to avoid bacterial growth.)

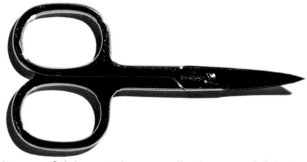

nail scissors - Quite useful in cutting small pieces of fabric, usually silk or linen, for nail wrapping and mending. Also popular for parents to groom children's nails.

emery boards - Select a variety of grades. Rough, coarse ones are good for shortening and shaping nails, especially acrylic. The finer ones are best for smoothing the nail edge, but not the plate. Leave that to the disk files and buffers.

disk files - Round, flat, flexible, and with many grades to choose from. They can bend easily, which makes them quite versatile. Especially good for removing ridges from the nail surface and smoothing it down, preparing it for buffing or polish.

polish remover pads - Lint-free pads that are perfect for removing products from the fingertips. Always fold pad onto itself and wipe nail with clean area.

(natural) cotton - For removal of varnish and other nail products. (Some synthetic "cottons," because of a lack of absorbency, tend to smear product more than remove it.)

white pencil - For use in whitening the underside of the nail and as a tracer when doing a "French" manicure. (Also a good, temporary way to keep the nail tips looking clean.)

orangewood stick (shown with plastic version) - For pushing back the cuticles and cleaning the nail surface. Especially effective in cleaning under the free edge and around the sides if the tip is covered with a bit of moistened cotton. Sometimes these are available with rubber-cushioned tips, which help to soften the pressure on the sensitive cuticles. (Avoid use of a metal instrument. The hardness of the tool can often break the skin and can do more harm than good.)

nail buffer (stick version) - For a beautiful, natural shine. Most sticks come with three working surfaces. The first area, usually one-half of one side and made of the coarsest material, is used to smooth out ridges and irregularities on the plate. The second, a finer grade, is meant to smooth out the plate even more and remove any tiny lines created by the first side. The final side, always grit-free, is meant solely for buffing. Buffing is very good for the circulation of blood underneath the nail and in the fingertip. (However, overbuffing can dry out the nail and create brittleness; use in moderation.)

nail stone (natural) - A natural pumice stone in the shape of a pencil. Best for removing excess bits of skin off the nail surface and around the cuticles.

toe separator - To keep the toes from touching one another when you are working on them. Indispensible if you like polishing your toenails. Better than using twisted bits of paper towel (the fibers can get into the polish).

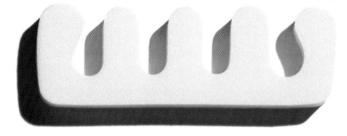

cuticle nippers - These are very precise instruments and should be used with caution. For clipping away only loose bits of skin **around** the cuticle (*Remember, you should not be removing the cuticle itself.*) They are best for cutting away only small pieces and should **never** be used to clip the nail itself. Doing so will dull the blades.

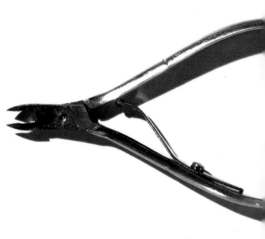

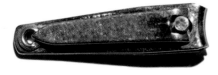

magnifying glass - This is essential for me to inspect my work, especially if the nails are going to be shown in a tight close-up photo. You need one only if your nails come under that much scrutiny.

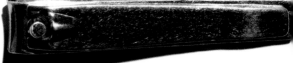

nail clippers (two versions) - I do not recommend the widespread usage of clippers, as they tend to bend the nail and weaken it. I prefer to maintain the shape by filing. However, they are very good for quick shortening of extralong nails. Just be sure to smooth out the small, sharp points that they create. The larger version is only for toenails, which should be cut straight across (and rounded at the sides).

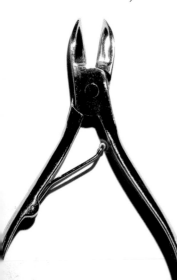

toenail scissors - Sometimes preferable to clippers because they cut through the toughened toenails with more ease. Always be sure to pull back the skin around the nail when cutting, to prevent an accidental cut. Good for clipping the sides of the toenail to prevent an ingrown nail.

nail brush - Good for cleaning the nails, especially underneath the free edge and around the cuticles. Very popular with men, but also used frequently by women. I prefer finer bristles that will not tear at the skin. Use with warm water and a mild soap. (*You can also try using a* **toothbrush**, *in a soft or fine texture, instead of the traditional brush. It will give you more control and is kinder to your fingers.*)

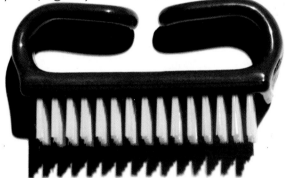

nail buffer (handheld) - This type of nail buffer is used often by men, although women use it as well. It gives you a quick, natural shine and the size and shape make it very easy to handle. The chamois or leather "cloths" should be replaced if the surface shows signs of wear. When you use a buffer, always sweep in one direction, away from the base of the nail. Lift the buffer off the surface after every movement to prevent "burning." (Overdoing it can dry out the nail and cause splitting.)

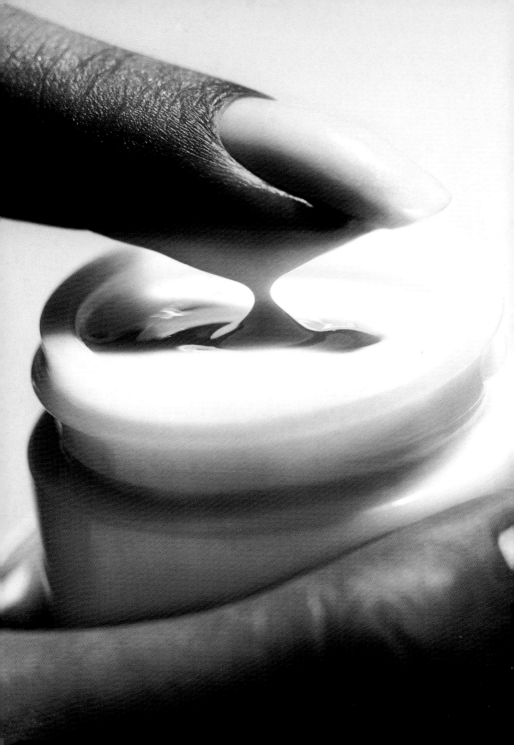

One trip to the cosmetics counter or your neighborhood drugstore should give you a good idea of just how many choices there are for nail care products, including everything from base coats to hardeners, cuticle cremes to nail varnishes. Here are just a few words of advice. Often, the ingredients for one manufacturer's product are identical to another's, but the pricing can be vastly different. In some instances what you may be paying for is great packaging and advertising. However, some of the best products on the market contain materials that do cost more. Ingredients that ensure better coverage, truer coloration, and longer wear may add to the price of your favorite brands.

Next time you go out shopping, take along the following list of products. It's made up of many of the things that I keep with me in both my professional *and* personal manicuring kits.

nail polish • **top coat** • **polish remover**
polish pen • **base coat** • **ridge filler**
buffing creme • **cuticle oil** • **cuticle creme**
moisturizer • **sealer** • **hardener** • **nail glue**
liquid or silk wrap • **nail art kit** • **decals**
acrylic nail kit • **nail tips** • **press-on nails**

Cuticle cremes are available in small pots like this one. Dab a little onto the ball of your fingertip, apply around the base of each fingernail, and massage in.

nail polish - Comes in a variety of shades and qualities, from sheer to metallic to cremes. Remember, they have a short shelf life and can dry out quickly.

top coat - To help protect polish from daily wear and tear.

polish remover - For removing polish and other products from the surface of the nail. (*Be sure to use one suited to your nails: dry, brittle, synthetic, etc.*)

polish pen - Good for removing excess polish from the sides of nails and to give a neater line around the cuticles.

base coat - A good one is usually a little thicker than a top coat and "sticky" enough to create a good base for your polish.

ridge filler - Goes on first, before anything, to create a smoother surface for base coats and polish.

buffing creme - Usually contained in small pots, dabbed onto nails to obtain a better shine when buffing.

cuticle oil - Just a little drop, massaged into the cuticle, helps nourish, moisturize, and keep it healthy-looking.

cuticle creme - Helps loosen and remove dead skin around the cuticle on the nail plate.

moisturizer - To add and prevent loss of moisture on the hands, feet, and nails.

sealer - Usually denser than a top coat. To seal and protect nail decorations, such as decals and paints.

hardener - Works directly on the surface of the nail to strengthen it.

nail glue - Used to apply nail tips or mend nails. Can also be used to apply decorations to nails.

liquid or silk wrap - Two quick ways to strengthen nails and to repair breaks and tears.

nail art kit - Usually contains decals and other decorations to create multicolored designs.

decals - Usually a variety of designs on multiple sheets.

acrylic nail kit - Multiple pieces, including foil templates, powders, and liquids to create your own nails.

nail tips - Plastic "half-nails" that come in a variety of sizes to fit every fingertip. Should be accompanied by nail glue.

press-on nails - Full plastic nails that are backed with double-sided adhesive. Come in a variety of sizes.

5 Nailed!

(The Basics of Nail Care)

Long nails are still, in some cases, highly sought after, but these days there are other options for achieving beautiful, yet practical, nails. Short or long, round or tapered, bright or subdued; they are all possibilities. The important thing is that whatever look you choose, you choose it wisely. Short, *unkempt* nails for a job where your hands show is just as inappropriate as long, colored nails when you need to perform intensive hand labor. Remember, your hands are an extension of you, and you can control what message they send out. Calling attention to your hands in the wrong way can backfire. But showing them to their best advantage creates an impression that reflects positively on you.

The first **basic** I want to address is overall good grooming for your hands (and feet). From when we are taught as children how to brush our teeth and comb our hair, I feel we should incorporate a bit of hand and foot grooming into our daily regimens. But don't worry, I am not advocating anything elaborate or difficult. Just something as simple as a little moisturizer massaged into the hand, then onto the nails and around the cuticles, and the same for the feet. This, I guarantee, will result in better groomed hands and feet that are virtually worry-free. Signs of age are quick to show up on our hands, but this little bit of pampering and care can easily offset them.

There are four main areas I take into consideration in deciding the final *look* a nail should have. They are **lifestyle, length, shape,** and **color** (see *chapter 6*). Before you do anything to your nails yourself, you should take into consideration *all* of these areas. I have also slipped cuticle care into this chapter because it is a "basic" too.

baby basics

Before we get too far along, I thought I'd give you some simple guidelines for tending babies' nails:
- Clip their nails while they are asleep; it's easier this way.
- Use scissors or baby clippers, but never shape the nails; clip straight across.(Also, gently pull away the fingertip to avoid an accidental cut.)
- Afterward, use a mild moisturizer (be sure to check ingredients) to keep the nails and hands forever soft.
- I know it might be tempting, but avoid using any nail products, such as polishes, as these may damage the structure of the nail plate.

Now on to more basics . . .

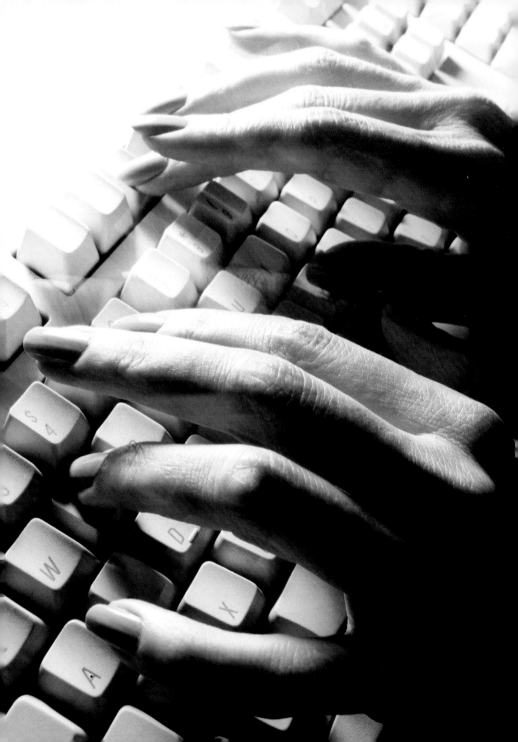

lifestyle

Women's roles have changed greatly over the years, and these changes have, undoubtedly, changed the way we look at ourselves. With a greater visibility in the workplace comes a respect for efficiency and practicality. As a result, we need to be more aware of our physical limitations and not let ourselves be handicapped by our grooming choices. Personally, I don't know if it's possible to type at a keyboard properly without running the risk of breaking or chipping a long nail. (*As a matter of fact, you should always be using the "pad" of your finger and not the nail tip itself if you want to prevent the tip breaking off.*)

However, there is no question that a saleswoman in a fashionable boutique should exercise the option to wear the latest in nail fashion. But even then she should think twice about a style that could interfere with the accomplishment of even the most mundane of tasks, such as working a cash register. Fortunately, some careers, such as those in entertainment, afford individuals the opportunity to be completely self-expressive. Interestingly, though, most of the top models I work with wear their nails short in order to remain versatile for a photo shoot or runway show.

Women (and men) are becoming increasingly aware of the grooming of their hands and nails, due in no small part to the huge popularity of personal computers.

length

How long you keep your nails is not just a question of looks, it is a question of appropriateness. If you have a job where long nails hinder the performance of your duties, then you should seriously consider keeping them short. If doing even the simplest of things, like dialing a phone or picking up an object from a desk, become long and drawn-out activities, you are seriously jeopardizing your ability to function properly. Besides, absolutely nothing is more infuriating than not being able to do something with your hands. In this workaday world, where time is money, extralong nails are a style few of us can afford. But for many, a long nail is the quintessence of femininity, a dramatic exclamation point for their personality. Cutting a nail grown long is like clipping Samson's hair; it removes a source of power. **This is beauty at its most psychological**. Many women still associate long nails with the privileged class and short ones with the working class. Yes, Barbra Streisand's nails are long and glamorous, but Oprah's are short and well groomed. Neither of them is the more influential because of her nail choice. Thankfully, there are lengths that fall somewhere in between that are quite beautiful and still practical.

There is no standard length that a nail should be; it depends on each individual. First, look at the length and shape of your

An "exaggerated" look at the length of a groomed nail.

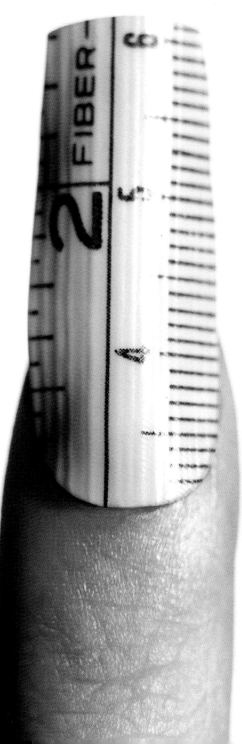

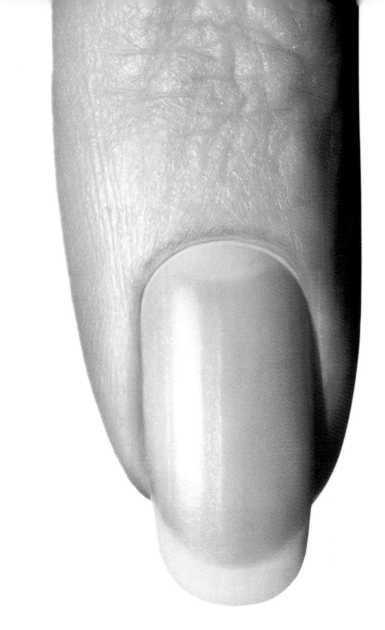

a perfectly shaped nail

fingers *and* hands. Personally, I feel the best length for a nail is one that naturally elongates the hands and fingertips, without exaggerating. For women with long, thin hands, adding too much in length can create a spidery, clawlike effect. Moreover, if your hands are round and fleshy, overly long nails can look misplaced. Much the same can be said of nails that are too short. Fingernails that end right at the free edge can look incomplete and stunted. Personally, I see nails that extend approximately 1/8″ to 1/4″ over the fingertip as a good starting measurement. I feel that this gives the fingertips just enough length to create elongation and gracefulness.

shape

Generally speaking, *my* favorite shape is one that mirrors the roundness of the nail at the base and cuticle. If done well, this is usually a pleasing oval shape that is not too tapered or square and looks quite natural. But the shape of the nail bed is not always oval. Sometimes the line extends almost straight across, other times it is a sharper curve. Regardless of what shape you have in mind, the first thing you need to do is work the nail edge down. Using the coarser side of an emery board, briskly rub along the free edge. Work from either side toward the center, going in **one** direction *straight out from the nail*, not inward, as this may cause it to fray. Once you have

My idea of the "perfect" nail. One that's not too long, with an edge that mirrors the shape at its base.

45

filed the nail down to its desired shape, smooth out the edge even more with a disk file. Then, with the disk, buff down any ridges on the plate. (This is necessary because ridge fillers can only do so much to even out the surface.) A glossy polish will intensify any marks, so you'll want to make the nail as smooth as possible. Remember though, when you are smoothing out the surface with a disk file you are removing layers of the nail. So don't overdo it, especially if you have thin nails already. Just take off the most obvious marks.

Some great shapes . . . .

. . . the **classic** *oval, perfect for any occasion . . .*

. . . an exotic, exaggerated **dagger** or **quill** shape, like the one I had the opportunity to create for Madonna in one of her videos . . .

. . . a simple yet elegant **pointed** tip, highlighted in white along with the lunula, was quite popular in the thirties . . .

. . . the extended square, a very "up-to-the-minute" look . . .

. . . and finally, a unique **notch**, created with precise filing.

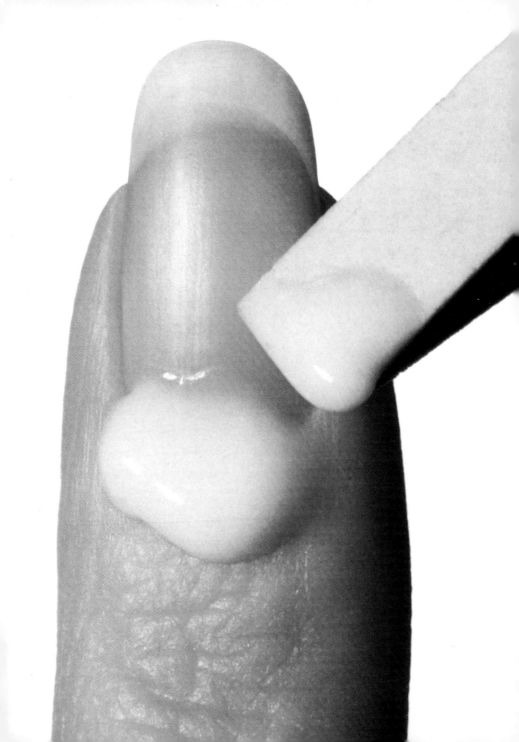

basic cuticle care

Many nail care specialists still disagree on the actual usefulness of a cuticle. As for myself, I believe it is there to help protect the nail bed from damage where it grows out from the fingertip. There was a time when most everyone thought it was best to clip cuticles away. This is not only obviously unneccessary, but potentially quite dangerous. It is very easy to cut into the skin and create a painful, infection-prone wound. But cuticles are apt to tear and rupture all on their own. This is especially the case if they are dry and brittle. If you find yours in this condition, I highly recommend that you get a professional to groom them into a workable state. Then, once they are back to normal, you yourself can follow the rest of these steps to maintain them.

First, massage a bit of cuticle creme (in some cases, cuticle remover) onto each cuticle and allow it to set for a few moments. Then, with an orangewood stick (never use metal, as it may tear at the skin), gently push back the cuticles. You should also use the stick, which you may want to cover in cotton and dip in antiseptic, to clean around the cuticle. (As an option, you may use a pointed nail stone, as seen in the picture opposite, to aid in the removal of any dead skin that remains on the nail plate.) Afterward, if you have any bits of

A bit of cuticle creme (or remover) massaged into the cuticle softens it and helps to remove dead skin. Using a pointed nail stone can be especially helpful for cleaning the surface of any debris.

torn cuticle remaining, you can clip them off with a pair of nippers. (Remember, though, a cuticle is there to protect the nail plate, and pieces should be cut only if they have split away.) Finally, wipe the nail surface clean with a piece of cotton moistened in antiseptic to remove any further debris, especially if you are planning to apply polish.

Whenever you have finished a basic manicure or an application of color, apply a touch of cuticle oil to each cuticle to keep it moist and healthy-looking.

Always groom your cuticles as part of your daily "beauty" routine.

Remember, in deciding matters of beauty and personal appearance, your favorite celebrity, current fashion trends, and even your friends can often influence your final choices. But try to keep them all at *arm's* length. Every set of hands (and nails) has its own guidelines, its own personal blueprint. If you know what you are working with, the answers are all right there.

Now that I've addressed all of these considerations, I have put together a simple, basic self-manicure that should work for any woman. . . .

Here is one example of a beautifully manicured hand.

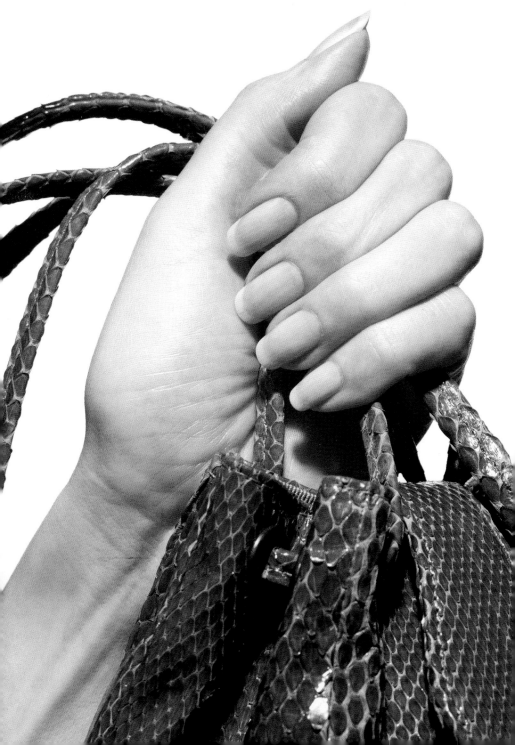

a seven-step

1

Remove any nail products from the surface of the nail. Dampen a cotton ball with remover and hold over the nail for a few seconds, then swipe *away from the cuticle (to avoid smearing polish).* Fold it over to get a clean area, redampen, and swipe again. Then, if necessary, dip an orangewood stick wrapped in a bit of cotton (or a swab) into remover to clean off any additional polish left on the nail plate.

2

Filing and shaping the nail. Using an emery board, tilted slightly under, work along the entire free edge. Work the file from side to center, side to center. Use quick, short strokes that move *away* from the nail, not into it. The edge should mirror the shape at the base. *Remember, never file nails when they are wet and most susceptible to damage.*

3

Smooth nail surface. For ridges, use a medium grade disk file over the area, lightly working back and forth. Use a fine grade to level and smooth even more. Clean the nail surface of loose debris. *Keep in mind, you're removing a layer of your nail, so don't overdo this step.*

4

Cuticles. Apply a generous amount of cuticle creme to each cuticle area and gently massage in. With an orangewood stick (wrapped in cotton), gently push the cuticle back from the nail plate. Rub off any bits of excess skin from the plate, sides, and grooves.

basic manicure

5

Clean tips. Wash your hands of all product and debris. Then, take a cotton-wrapped orangewood stick, dipped in solvent, and work around the underside of each free edge, applying gentle pressure from the center to the sides. Then, trace along the edge with a white manicuring pencil in the same manner. (This is especially good for a temporary whitening effect and "French" manicure look.)

6

Buffing the nails. Once you've smoothed out the nails, it's your choice whether to polish, "French" manicure, decorate, or leave the nails clean. If you choose the latter, take a buffer and gently work all over the nail surface in a horizontal (side-to-side) motion. If you are too vigorous, you'll feel a burning sensation. This is a sign that you are applying too much pressure and drying out the nail. Go easy, and lift the buffer off the nail plate after every stroke. (*You can, if you like, add polish after buffing your nails.*)

7

Application of moisturizers and cuticle oils. After buffing, and as a finishing touch if you choose not to add polish, take a favorite moisturizer (personally, I prefer specially formulated nail oils) and work into and around the entire nail area, including the cuticles. This will help prevent breakage, splitting, and damage due to dryness and abuse, especially if you decide not to wear polish.

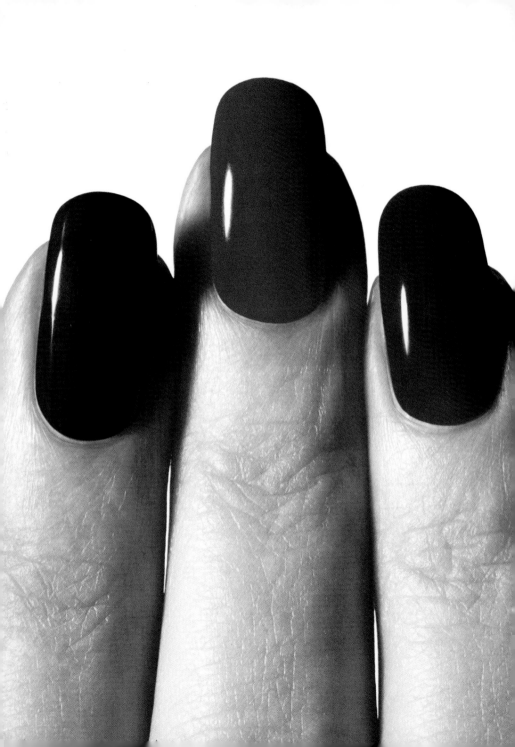

6 A Show of Hands!

(Color and Special Techniques)

This is the chapter where we get to have a little fun and be adventuresome. A person should only be limited by his or her imagination when it comes to beauty choices. However, without trying intentionally to dampen your spirits, a bit of the practical should always be a part of the overall picture. Lengths, styles, and colors change so quickly sometimes that there seems to be a new hot idea out there before your polish has a chance to dry. And even though we all like to keep up with the latest things, consistency is the true hallmark of great personal style. After saying all of this, I hope you don't think I wouldn't want you to try something new. Not at all! Just a bit of common sense, sprinkled with your enthusiasm, is my two cents' worth of advice!

> **Color choices can optically change the appearance of a nail's shape. For instance, a deep red color on a square-shaped nail will make it look wider. A pale color on the same nail will make it seem longer.**

A trio of richly colored nails, all variations of red.

In this chapter I'll talk about a variety of what I consider "special techniques." Incidentally, I placed color polish application in this section because it needs more attention than a basic manicure and requires a certain amount of upkeep to maintain its good looks. So on the next few pages we'll talk about:

a modified "French" manicure

synthetic nails:
tips, acrylics, and press-ons

color polish application

decal application

nail painting

stones and glitter

ring application

Here is an example of my modifed "French" manicure. As you can see, the tips are still prominent, but not distractingly so..

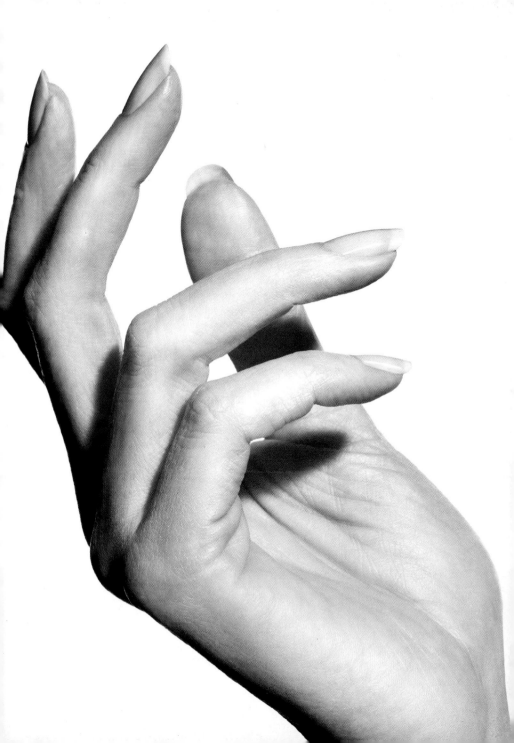

1. Take a white pencil and emphasize the underside of the free edge for a better guide.

2. Then, with a white or off-white polish, arc across the fingertips.

(Incidentally, a dark-colored polish with a white tip is not a French manicure. If you want this look, first apply two coats of your colored polish, then apply the arcs of white. Over that, apply a clear top coat for protection.)

3. After the arcs have dried, apply first one, then a second coat of sheer polish, all over the nail.

4. Add a third coat of clear polish, for added protection.

58

a modified "French" manicure

Personally, I think the contrast between a white, white tip and flesh-colored plate in a basic "French" manicure is too strong, so my modified version follows the same steps, but utilizes softer coloring to create a subtler feeling, without sacrificing the desired effect.

The first step is to give yourself a basic manicure all the way to the end. Next, take white (or off-white) polish and apply in an "arc" across the top of each nail. You can, if you want, use your eye and the actual nail edge as a guide. But there are strips of tape made expressly for this purpose, and they can be a great help. (*You can also give yourself a better guide by first using a white pencil underneath the free edge.*) Next, use the flesh-colored **sheer** polish to paint the entire nail, even *over* the white tip. This first coat will subtly change the color of the white. By the second coat, you will be able to see a marked difference. The tip is not nearly as harsh, but is still noticeable. You can go onto a third, clear top coat to seal and protect.

For a variation, try painting the lunula white along with the tip. This particular version was quite popular in the 1930s, and has continued to pop up on stylish hands ever since.

synthetic nails: tips, acrylics, and press-ons

What's amazing about all the choices we have today as consumers is that if you don't like what you have naturally, you can always go out and buy something to replace it. Sometimes the replacement is even better than the original. Certainly this is true of some nail care products. If you have short, brittle nails, you are only a box away from hard, durable ones. Want a fancy stone-applied tip tonight, but need to go to work tomorrow without it? It's yours with one quick stop at the cosmetics counter. But these products are not without their drawbacks. Too much usage can actually damage and weaken the real nail underneath. So use a bit of caution when you work with them.

Tips, like the one shown in our "X-ray" photo opposite, are quite popular and simple to apply. In what is sometimes referred to as a "half-nail" application, glue is run along the translucent band and the tip is adhered directly to the free edge of the real nail. After the glue has had a moment to dry, a coat of acrylic "overlay" is painted over the entire nail, tip and all. This will cover over the thin seam created by the tip and make for a smoother nail surface. (All materials should be included in a tip kit.) Once the nail has dried, you can file and apply polish as desired. An **acrylic nail** is created with a small amount of synthetic powder mixed with liquid and spread

Notice three things in our nail tip "X-ray": the number at the top showing the size of the tip; the lighter arc area, which is the part to be glued down; and the free edge of the real nail itself, where the tip is adhered.

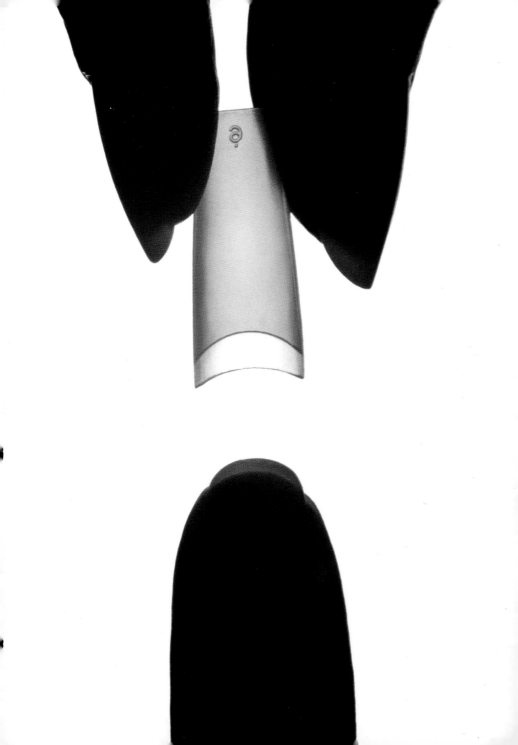

1. First, place the foil template under the free edge of a manicured nail. (Be sure that it is level with the real nail.) Affix by pressing adhesive areas to sides of the finger.

acrylic basics

2. After dipping brush into powder and liquid ingredients, forming a small ball, dab right onto the area where the free edge overhangs the template. Brush outward **only**, along the sides, and onto the template.

4. For coat number three, redip and apply onto the **back** of the nail. (This can be the **wettest** application.) Be careful not to disturb the cuticle. Brush to the sides and outward all the way to the edge of the newly created nail. 5. Allow time to dry and gently remove template. 6. File and shape as you would a real nail.

3. For coat two, redip the brush and this time dab onto the **middle** of the nail plate, smoothing to the sides and outward only.

62

over the nail with a brush. (Again, all materials should be included in their own kit.) There is a special foil template that you place under the free edge of your nail so you can extend the acrylic to the desired length. Once an acrylic nail has dried and the template is gently pulled away, it can be handled in exactly the same manner as a real nail. This type of technique is recommended for women who want a longish look but have nails that are brittle or weak. **Press-on nails** are the easiest of all to apply, but I would recommend them only if you have no other options, as they are not very resilient. They are purchased in sizes, similar to tips, and are attached using double-sided adhesive strips, which are usually included with the nails.

One very important thing to watch out for: That you (or your nail technician) not leave any air space between the real and the synthetic nail, as this can trap moisture and encourage bacterial growth. (Unfortunately, this is an especially frequent occurrence with acrylics.) You can discourage this if you first make sure to remove all products from the nail plate and lightly sand the entire surface with a disk file to aid in the complete adhesion of the product.

I also strongly suggest seeking the assistance of a professional manicurist to **remove** a synthetic nail. Even though there are products available for at-home use, you can avoid the possibility of tearing, breaking, or damaging the real nail underneath by getting help from a professional.

Most special techniques require that your color polish be applied before they are done. So here is a simple five-step procedure. First, all products, such as oils, cremes, and removers, should be thoroughly cleansed from the nail surface. Otherwise, the polish will not adhere properly.

Step One

Filing the nail. Check the nail surface for any pronounced ridges, bumps, or marks. Using a disk file, lightly smooth out the entire nail, paying close attention to the cuticle area and softening any sharp edges. (Sharp edges increase the risk of chipping.)

Step Two

Applying the base coat. I recommend a base coat (or ridge filler). It smooths out the surface even more and helps the polish adhere better and last longer. Apply the base coat in the same manner as polish, but only one coat is necessary. Allow time to dry.

Step Three

Applying polish. First, be sure that the polish is mixed properly, as it tends to separate. When applying polish, do so in quick, light strokes. Apply the dipped brush to the very center of the nail first, then sweep once along both sides, so that you avoid having any excess polish running into the nail grooves. (Try not to get polish on the underside of the free edge. A lot of us have the habit of picking at our nails, and polish under the tip adds to the chances of it chipping and being pulled off the plate). When you go on to the next nail, always redip your brush, as polish dries quickly and can end up streaking. Apply two coats.

Over time some polishes can discolor the nail plate, so when selecting a polish, always look to see if it has a nonyellowing formula. This goes for base coats too.

color polish

With a sheer polish, always wait until the first coat is absolutely dry, or else the second coat can cause a striping effect.

Step Four

Removing excess polish. Dip an orangewood stick into polish remover and gently swipe around the edges of the nail, the grooves, the cuticles, and the underside. Redipping the stick as you go along will dissolve any polish you pick up. (You can use a pointed cotton swab. However, it can leave little fibers along the nail.)

Step Five

Applying a top coat. A top coat is great for added protection and can enhance the **shine** of your polish. Usually one coat is sufficient and is applied in the same manner described in step three.

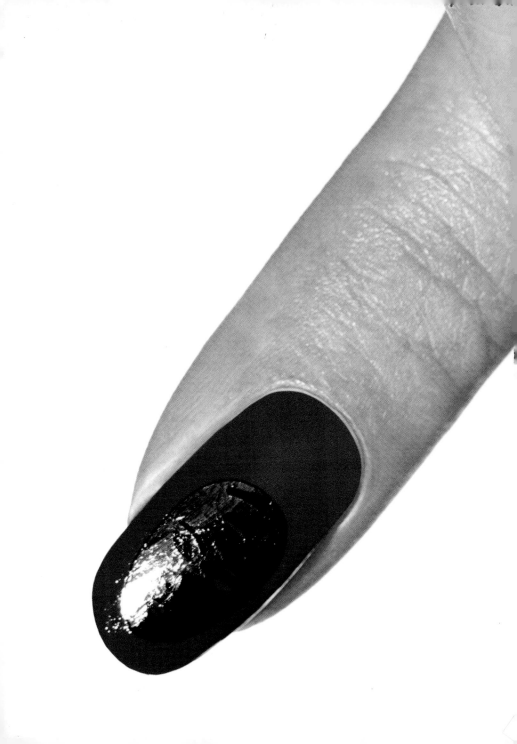

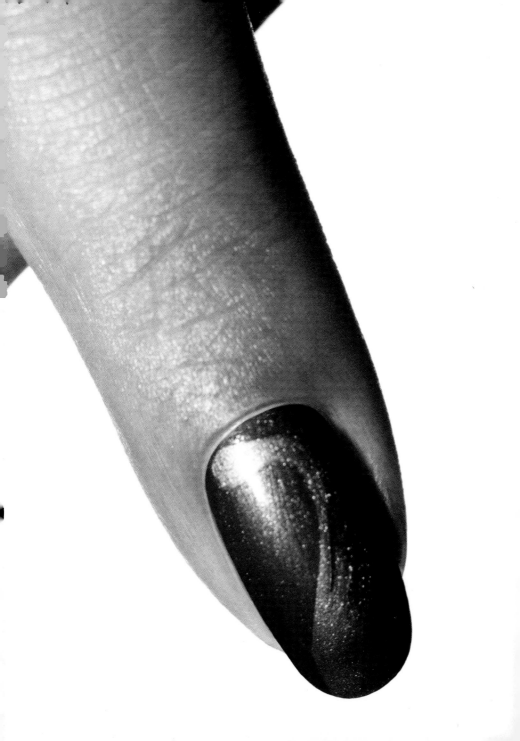

decals

One of the most popular types of nail art is a decal. Decals are available in a huge variety of designs and are very easy to apply. There are three common types of decals. The first, as seen on page 66, is applied after soaking the piece (which is clipped from the rest on a sheet) in water, then sliding it onto a dry, clean nail. The second is adhesive-backed. The third, usually a foil design, needs a special emulsifier to adhere properly to the nail. In all three instances, using a pair of tweezers can help you to accurately place the design. Some decals are quite fragile and can practically disintegrate before your eyes, especially if you play around with them too long before setting them on the nail.

A few other things to watch out for:

• Always make sure the nail surface is free and clear of debris and product, unless, of course, you are applying the decal over a polished nail.

• Be sure there are no air bubbles trapped under the surface, as that will increase the chances of chipping.

• A sealer should be applied for added protection; this is denser than the usual clear top coat.

• Your nail polish should be completely dry before you try to place your decal or you can easily damage or mar the surface.

nail painting

There are two ways you can paint on the surface of the nail. One is to create a design freehand, like what I have done for the photo (on page 67), or you can use the airbrushing equipment and stencil techniques necessary to create more elaborate designs. The first is, of course, somewhat easier because you can do it yourself, but you do need a steady hand. The second application is best left up to a professional manicurist or artist.

How I created my example of nail painting was very simple. I started with a base color, which is sometimes called a master color, and **painted** a curlicue on top of it. (If you want to paint finer lines and details, you can work with a real **art brush**, instead of a nail brush like I did. Just be sure that it can be used with nail polishes and solvents.) The direction of this design is from the cuticle down to the free edge, but designs are frequently seen going the other way. Also, I used similarly toned colors, to create a softer, subtler feel. (Contrasting colors, besides sometimes being quite bright, can point up inaccuracies in application.) Most nail-art paint is water-based, so mistakes can easily be corrected and removed from the skin, but you can also use polish, as I did. Last, I finished with a clear sealer to protect the artwork.

(Incidentally, nail-art designs hold better on an acrylic nail than on a real one.)

stones and glitter

A stone is always applied **after** your color polish and top coat. Flatter, smaller stones can be imbedded into the polish right before drying is complete. That way they can sink in and become almost flush with the rest of the surface. Larger stones, however, don't benefit as much from this. It is easiest to use nail glue when applying a stone. (You may use a stronger cement to prevent the stone from breaking off.) Whatever adhesive you use, only a drop is necessary. Finally, I do not recommend using a top coat over a stone, because it can dull the sparkle.

Glitter, the way you see it shown here, was applied separately, right on top of a coat of olive green polish. First, I took a clean nail brush and dipped it into a clear gloss top coat, and then into the glitter (which came in its own small container). Then I painted right on the colored nails. This was followed by an additional clear top coat to prevent any particles from flaking off. (Applying glitter this way will give a free-form effect to the glitter and create more sparkle than using polish that already contains metallic bits, because you are typically adding more.)

Here is a triple combination of unusual elements: olive green base polish, opalescent glitter in clear coat, and a large, yellow rhinestone (always use a crystal one for the best sparkle).

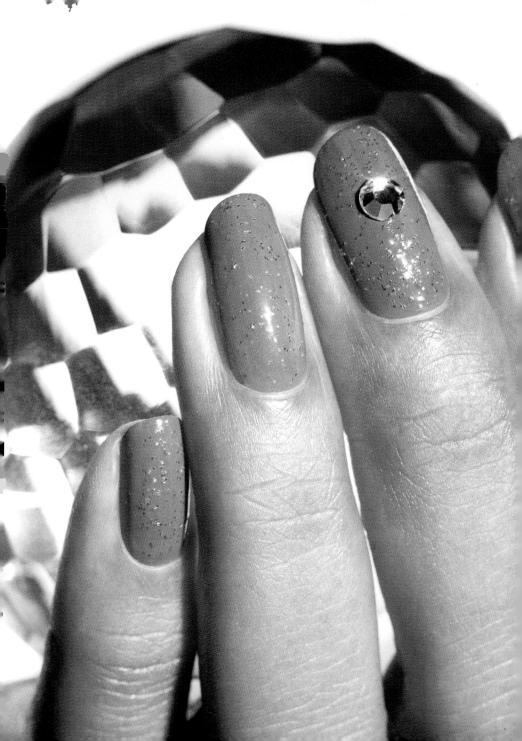

ring application

This is a rather unorthodox form of nail decoration, but after the response I received from doing it in a beauty magazine, I decided to include it here. However, I recommend that you have a professional do this on a synthetic nail, preferably a nail tip. Professionals have the proper equipment, including a manicuring drill.

First, taking a felt marker, dot a spot on the unattached synthetic nail where you know the ring will hang freely. Next, use an awl, circle compass (like the one's you used in school), or paper clip to make the hole itself. The most effective way to do this is by applying a bit of heat to the tip of either implement. (You can do it without it, but the hole you create will probably not be wide enough to accommodate the ring.) Heat the tip sufficiently so that it will melt through the plastic nail. (A lit match is a suitable heat source.) Poke through the top of the nail first, at the marked spot, then through from the bottom. (*Be sure to cover over the table surface you are working on to avoid scratches.*) All this should take only a few seconds; do not linger over the nail. Give it a moment to cool down, then adhere the tip to the real nail. File down any bumps or ridges and polish as usual. Finally, place the ring into the hole. You can use anything, even an earring, just be sure to watch the ends, so that they don't accidentally scratch the surface of the polish.

Here a silver ring is hanging from extralong, square-tipped acrylic nails polished in a beautiful gunmetal color.

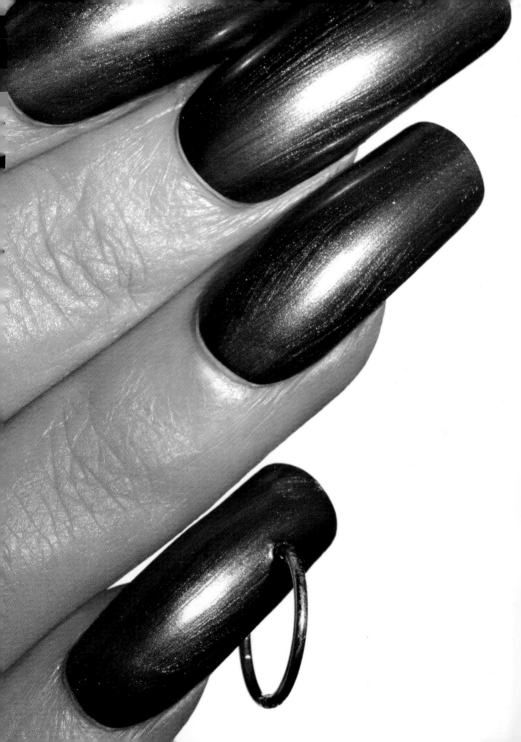

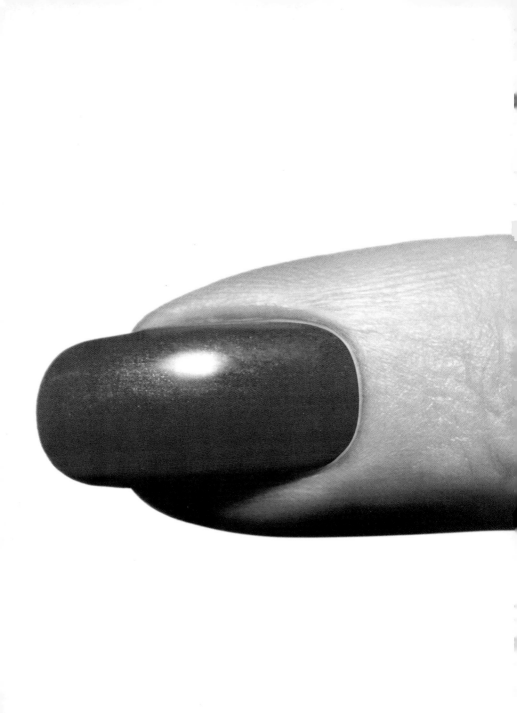

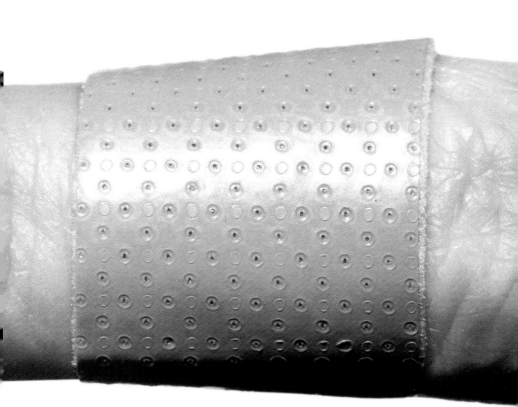

7 Hands Off!
(Nail Care First Aid)

One of the least glamorous, but nonetheless necessary, parts of my business is taking care of nail problems. And unfortunately, they come up much more often than you might think. Models are constantly showing up on the set with hangnails, broken tips, chipped polish, and, sometimes, much worse. Mostly, these problems stem from neglect or abuse. Either way, there are some good and fast ways to mend and alter the nail surface, thus preventing many of these problems from returning. However, severely damaged or diseased nails should never be treated by yourself or a manicurist. In these instances, I urge you to consult a doctor. Delay and avoidance will only serve to worsen the condition. Still, there is some nail damage that, with the right instruction, you can attend to on your own. Solutions can be short- or long-term. And, if you don't already have them in your bathroom cabinet, you'll need to get two things: antibiotic ointment and antiseptic. These simple household products are amazing healers and preventatives.

The dreaded, painful hangnail is usually caused by excessive dryness or careless removal or unnecessary cutting of the cuticles. When these things occur, the cuticle can split away from the nail. It is also a very easy way to get an infection because your hands come in such constant contact with dirt, grime, and germs. It's best to always keep the cuticle pushed back with an orangewood stick. However, if you already have a hangnail, the first thing you should do is gently trim away any and **only** the excess skin. Then apply a dab of antibiotic ointment. **It is most important to keep the area soft and supple, to prevent further breaks**. In most cases, you should also keep varnishes and other products away from the cut. Just to be safe, if you want to wear a polish, it should be applied away from the immediate area.

The fungus among us!

A few ways to prevent or inhibit the growth and spread of nail fungus and infections:

- Apply a fungicidal creme to the nail plate between applications of synthetic nails.
- Make sure there is no **air space** between the real and the synthetic nail, especially acrylics, as this can trap moisture and breed fungus.
- Wear sandals in **wet areas** of gyms, public pools, etc.
- Wipe **antiseptic** between and around the sides and cuticles of the toes to kill bacteria-causing germs.
- **Always** make sure all tools and implements are properly cleaned (or sterilized) before using.

broken or split nails

Typically, a broken or split nail occurs for one or more of these reasons: an accident, carelessness, or weakness or brittleness of the nail. I can't give much advice to the careless or accident-prone, except to be more alert and watch out! But for those who have nails that break easily because of weakness, here's a bit of commonsense advice: Length plays an important part, so it is best to keep nails as short as you are comfortable with, because obviously the longer they are the more susceptible to breakage they become. Furthermore, the only way to truly strengthen the nails is with applications of nail oils and hardeners, and, most important, proper nutrition. Once a break or tear has occurred, the first thing to do is assess the amount of damage. Different levels of harm will need different levels of repair.

With a torn or split nail, look to see how far down the free edge it has occurred and then to see if there was any excess damage done to either side of the tear. It is also a good time to decide if you want to cheat and just trim away the damaged nail and repolish. Your only sin will be making one nail shorter than the rest. If the tear is minimal and the halves match up, the fix is relatively simple. First, remove all polish, then squeeze a bit of nail glue onto the nail surface. (Let the glue set for a moment, to get tacky.) Next, hold for a few moments, using gentle pressure. Then reapply the glue and add a piece of tissue, silk wrap, or fiber mender, to cover the area. Allow to dry. Last, using a disk file, buff the nail to smooth the surface and, if you like, reapply any polish.

When a tear has occurred *into* the nail bed, you must first clean the area of all products. But be careful; polish remover should not go into a cut. Once the area is cleansed, use antiseptic to kill any bacteria. Allow the nail to properly air dry. Personally, I would recommend applying medicated ointment to the cut and leaving it alone until it heals. (In most cases, this will only take a couple of days.) Then you can think about reapplying any nail polish.

Along with the antiseptic and antibiotic, nail glue is the most important product to have around the house for repairing the nail yourself. And although nail "extenders" are mainly used to lengthen the nail, they can also be partially effective in treating damage. If you have broken or split an artificial nail, it is best that you have a professional manicurist mend it because you can easily make the damage worse or more noticeable.

Don't go near the water!

*Even though soaking your hands and feet will soften the nails, **never** file or cut them while they are wet (or even moist). When the nail has absorbed moisture, the fibers expand slightly and become more pliable. That makes them much more susceptible to tearing and other damage.*

Also, try not to use a metal file or cuticle pusher, as these instruments are too rough on the nail. An emery board and an orangewood stick are much more flexible.

weak nails

Unfortunately, for people with weak nails the solutions are mainly topical. Nail hardeners (and strengtheners), when applied on the nail **plate**, have only a short-term effect because the nail's outer cells are already dead. *It is much the same with hair and hair care products.* However, for a more long-term solution, a change in diet may help, because your health does affect the appearance and strength of your nails.

Nail wrapping is a technique that also can be helpful for people who suffer from weak nails. (They're also good for quick fixes and adding length.) Nail wrapping uses silk, sometimes linen and other fabrics, which, when cut into small pieces, are glued directly onto the nail surface. They can be reinforced with glue, and, once they are dry, smoothed down for polish application.

For some, a "liquid wrap" is an even easier method to strengthen the nails. Liquid wraps contain small bits of fiber in a liquid form similar to polish. Liquid wraps are especially good for quick repairs of broken nails.

There are quite a few different ways to fix chipped polish and avoid redoing the whole nail, but most take a little practice. One in particular is *my* quick way to repair a chip. Try it out for size:

You'll need your remover and your polish. First, take the pad of your fingertip and moisten with remover. Quickly swipe across the chipped area. While you're cleaning off the remover from the pad of your finger, the polish around the chip should be softened. Now, take some polish on your polish brush and dab it right onto the chip and let it set for a few seconds. (This wait is necessary to "build-up" the coats that were stripped away). Then immediately put a coat of polish over the entire nail. If this is done correctly you shouldn't be able to see any lines. And it shouldn't take more than a minute or two, once you've mastered the technique.

To clean up smudges, you can use remover on a cotton swab, but be careful that loose fibers don't get into polish that hasn't had a chance to dry. (Try using a pointed swab, for more accuracy.) Personally, I like to use an orangewood stick, dipped in the remover. This way, I have much more control and can get smoother lines. Also, when I dip the stick back into the remover, I instantly dissolve any polish that was picked up on the stick and I don't have to worry about smearing it around the finger.

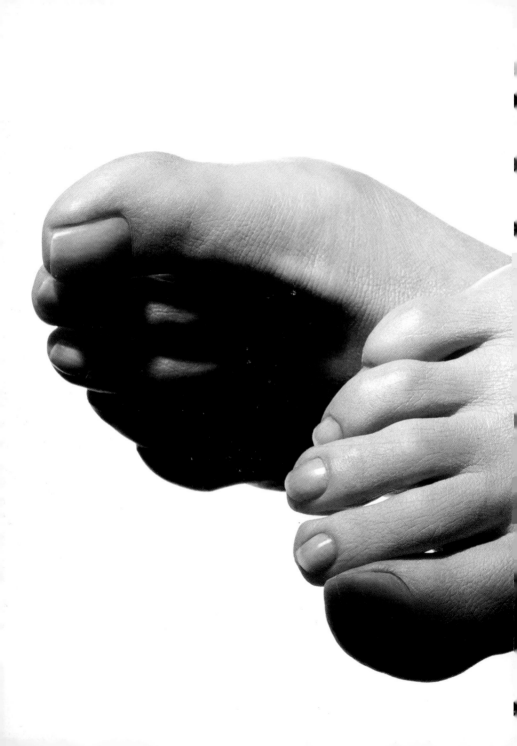

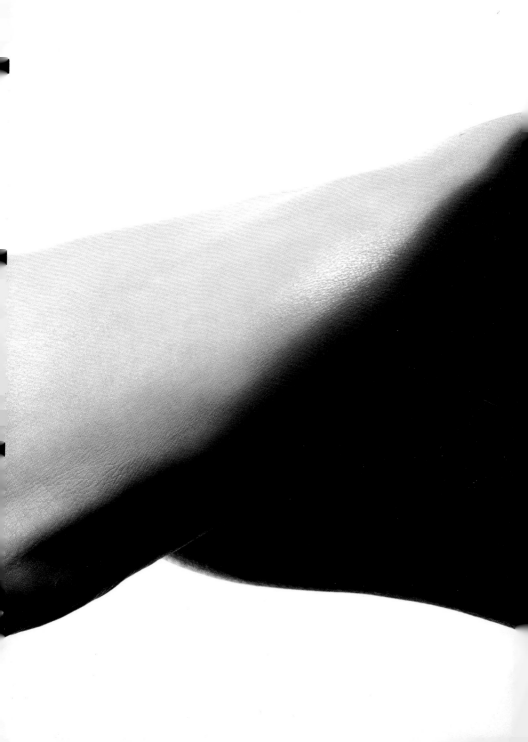

8 Best Foot Forward

(Foot Care)

Amazingly, many of us will spend a great deal of time, effort, and money on the care of our face and hands, while the feet go sorely unattended. It's really a shame, considering how easy it is to maintain them. Maybe because they are covered up much of the time, they are easily forgotten. You know, "out of sight, out of mind." But push them too far and the neglect and abuse can really start to show. There is nothing more unattractive than feet with heavily callused heels and toes and unkempt nails, especially when they are revealed in a beautiful pair of slippers or sandals. Furthermore, your feet take a lot of pounding and pressure; they need some pampering and care to recover and function properly. Moreover, working on your toenails is pretty much the same as working on your fingernails, with one major **positive** difference; you'll have the use of both your hands to do the tending! So with a simple reorganization of your daily "beauty" routine, pretty feet can and will be yours!

The following is a simple multistep pedicure that includes color polishing and a little bit of "massage therapy." Your feet have never had it so good!

Previous page: A pair of beautiful bare feet, after a simple pedicure.
Right: Classically manicured toes colored with light, neutral glitter polish.

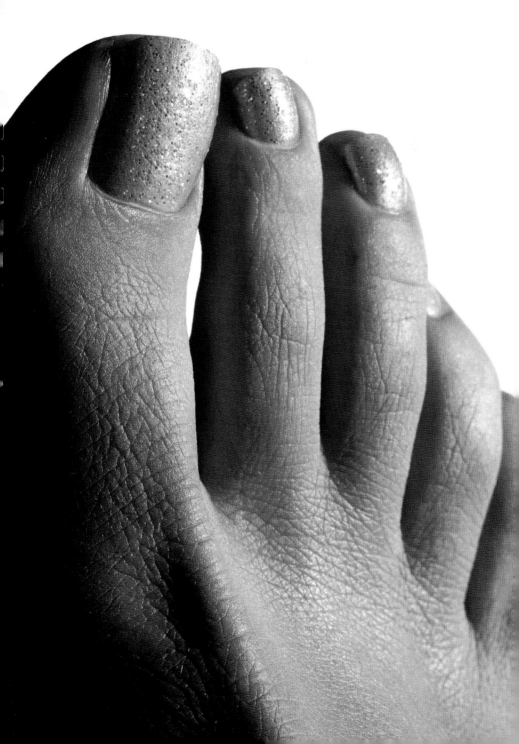

a perfect pedicure

shaping

The first thing you need to do is work on the nails themselves. Take a pair of toenail scissors and cut the nails straight across, leaving just a bit of free edge and slightly rounded sides (to avoid getting an ingrown nail). *When you use a pair of scissors, be sure to pull the skin back as you cut, to prevent accidental nipping of the skin.* Then file and smooth down the edges. (This way, you'll diminish the chances of running your hose.) If you have some noticeable ridges or bumps on the surface of the toenails, now is also the time to smooth them out. Take a disk file and lightly work over the surface, only removing what is necessary. However, in some cases, there will be **measurable** build-up of the nail on some toes, especially the pinkies. For this you can use a medium-grade disk file to briskly rub it down to a manageable thickness.

cleaning

Next, run some water in the tub and soak your feet. You can add foot salts to the water. *These are intended to make the surface of the skin softer and aid in the removal of callused and dried skin, especially around the heels and toes.* For light build-up of dead skin, use of a sloughing creme should be effective. Excess build-up is best removed by using a hand-held pumice stone. (When using pumice stones, always go gently in a circular motion over the surface. Don't try to make up for lost time by being overaggressive with hardened skin. Rubbing too roughly can cause injury.) If you attend to your feet regularly in this way, you should see results in a very short amount of time. I do not recommend trying to remove calluses or build-up with a cutting tool, by either yourself or a manicurist. They should be taken off by a podiatrist. (If you plan to take a

86

shower or bath, you might want to do so first, before shaping the nails and working the cuticles. However, always allow for the toenails to dry thoroughly before you trim them. Filing or cutting a nail when it is moist can easily cause damage or injury.)

cuticles

Now place a bit of cuticle creme on all the cuticles and massage in. Take a pointed nail stone and gently push back the cuticles. At the same time, rub off any excess dead skin from the surface of the nail and out of the grooves. (Here, I prefer using a nail stone to an orangewood stick because the build-up on the toes can be denser than on the fingers, and may need stronger measures.) After you're finished with all the toes, clean them off with a hand towel, rubbing briskly.

moisturizing

Now take moisturizer and rub all over the feet, especially into the drier areas around the heels and on any calluses. Avoid getting moisturizer in between the toes, as this excess moisture can breed germs. Take a cotton-wrapped orangewood stick, dipped in antiseptic, and wipe around the surface of the nail, especially around the cuticles, in the nail grooves, and under the free edge, to clear out debris and kill fungus-breeding germs and bacteria. Then take a cotton ball, also dipped in antiseptic, and work in between the toes. Last, if there are any loose bits of skin around the nail or cuticle, this is the only time I would say to use a nipper.

polish

Follow the same steps to put polish on the toes as you would the fingers. Always be sure to give the polish sufficient time to dry, as it is easy to mar or dent the surface of a nail when you put your feet into socks or shoes. If you choose not to wear polish at all, take a tiny bit of nail oil and rub it onto the surface of the nail and cuticle to keep them healthy and soft. (Remember, use just enough oil to keep the cuticle moist. **Don't flood the nail.** A little will go a long way.)

massage

There is some question about the real health benefits of a massage, but honestly, nothing feels better. After a hard day's work, a good rub can stimulate the circulation, ease tension, and increase flexibility.

A massage is usually most effective if done after a manicure or pedicure. Using massaging oils, apply a dime-size portion into each palm, then onto the area you are massaging. Try not to use too much, as this will feel more slippery than soothing. Then, using the balls of your fingertips, rub in a circular motion all over the foot (or hand). Try to apply the emphasis on the area at the center of the bottom of the foot (as pictured here) and around the heels, and do the same with the palms of the hands. Always try to move downward, not upward. From the ankle to the toes, from the wrists to the fingertips. Pull and stretch at the muscles and joints more than you push. However, it is not recommended that you deliberately try to "crack" any joints, although this may occur naturally. Try extending the massage up to the ankles, calves, and knees, when working on the feet, and up to the elbow, including the wrist and forearm, when working the hands. (Stress and tension are connected to these immediate areas). When you are finished, wipe away excess oils to prevent any accidents, and, if you like, dust on a bit of powder (or antiseptic) onto the feet.

A massage is the perfect finale to a great pedicure.

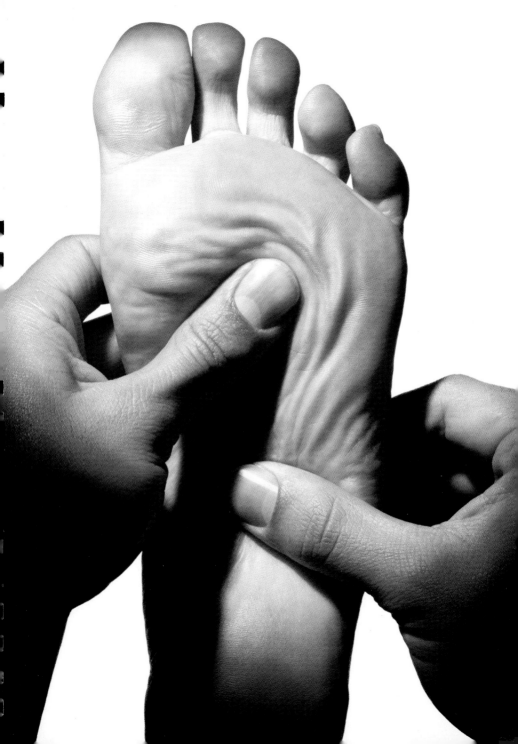

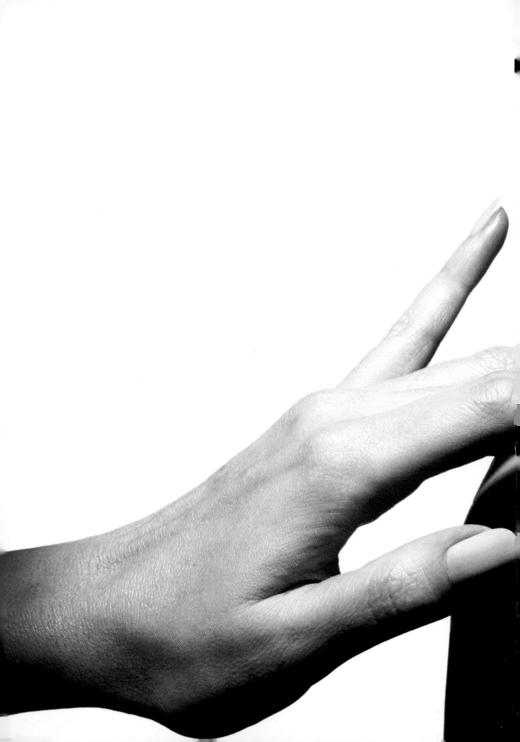

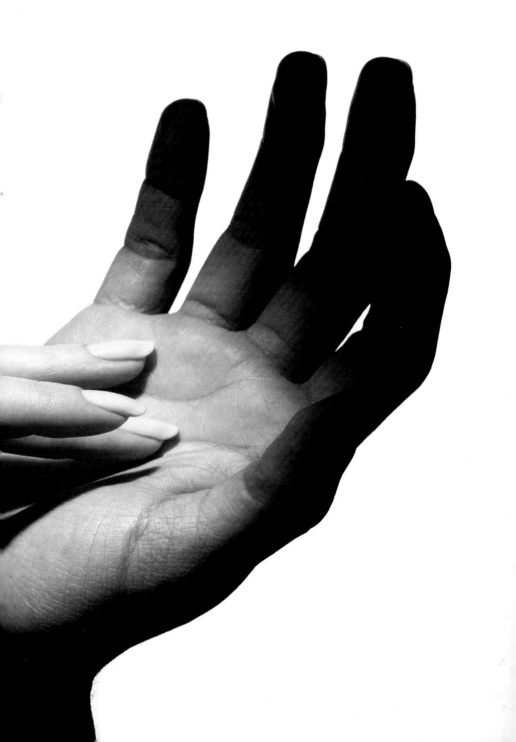

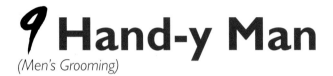

9 Hand-y Man
(Men's Grooming)

I know that for many men nail care consists of washing the hands (hopefully, with soap) and clipping nails periodically, usually over a wastebasket (if one is handy). To them, nail care is a matter of habit. When we are young we're taught about proper hygiene and grooming. Hopefully, as we get older, we continue to practice them, but somewhere along the way some of you guys got side-tracked. The word "dirt" became synonymous with "boy," and the two have cohabitated ever since. Furthermore, for you, the idea of a manicure or even simple nail grooming is too pretentious or effete. Certainly not a manly endeavor. However, if your habits are good ones (and you know which ones are and which aren't) you can skip ahead. If they're not, then continue reading. For those of you who are still with me, I know you're thinking that if I can tell you what to **do** in the next five minutes or less, then yes, maybe you'll consider it. But nothing more than that! Further, if the steps take **longer** than five minutes, forget it! I've taken all this into consideration and here is my four-part solution:

file-clean-moisten-buff

Previous spread: Men and women should treat their nails with the same care and attention. Right: A "typical" man's hand, in a "typical" pose?

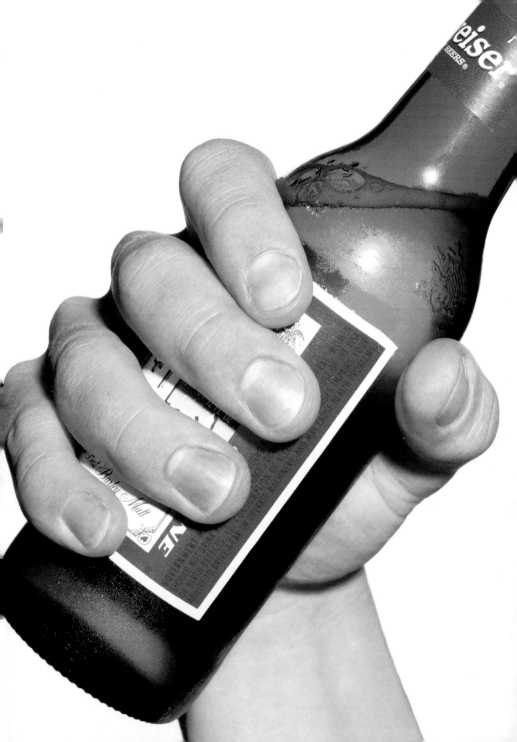

If it's been a long time since you've properly groomed your nails, this may take more than five minutes. However, once you get them back to a presentable state, it shouldn't take any time at all.

file

Now, I know most of you guys don't have a nail file, so you may have to go out and get one. Clipping is okay, but only to get the nails to a manageable length, then you'll still need the file to smooth the edges. If you maintain them, you will eventually be doing less clipping *and* less filing.

Cut the nail across and slightly rounded at the sides. The free edge should only be about a sixteenth of an inch long. Then, with the file, smooth out the edges created by the clipper. Work from side to center to side. Filing at a slight angle *under* the nail edge should help to clean it up too.

clean

Take a nail brush (*if you don't have one you should get one*) and with some soap and warm water, gently scrub all around the nails. The bristles of the brush should be firm enough to remove dirt, but soft enough not to tear at the skin. Be especially sure to clean around the cuticles and under the free edge. Dry your hands and fingers thoroughly. If you wish, you can take a white pencil and add emphasis under the free edge.

moisten

Take a bit of hand moisturizer and apply it to the cuticles. Then, with an orangewood stick (which you may not have) or, at least, one of your other fingernails, gently push the cuticle back off the nail. Simultaneously, you should also clean excess bits of skin with the stick, or your nail, from the surface. (Most of this should have been removed already with cleaning.) When you've finished all your cuticles, rub any remaining moisturizer into the fingers. Add more moisturizer, especially around the places where there is dryness, such as the knuckles and calluses.

buff

Use either a handheld or stick buffer and work horizontally (side to side) across each nail, being sure to get the sides and around the cuticle. Do not overbuff, as this will dry out the nail and make it brittle. If the nail is getting hot, you're doing it too hard. Here, the use of a buffing creme comes in handy, and increases the shine. When you're finished your nails will have a great natural look. I feel that this is preferable to wearing a clear polish, but it is your call. If you do wear polish, be sure it is a nonyellowing formula (this goes for clear or colored), as some men's nails can discolor over time, especially if you compound the risk by smoking.

for the feet

Most men won't take the time to file their toenails, but try at least using an emery board to smooth out any excess build-up on the nails, especially on the smaller toes. You should also consider using a pumice stone along the rough areas of your feet, including the sides and around the heel. This is especially easy right after a shower. (*Remember, never* **file** *your nails when they are wet!*)

Toenails should be cut straight across, with the edges clipped diagonally at the sides, to prevent an ingrown nail. Moisten and push back your cuticles, using an orangewood stick (or pointed nail stone) and moisturizer. Then apply more moisturizer to dry spots, such as calluses and heels, but clean up any excess, especially in between the toes, where bacteria can breed. Then, add a light dusting of foot powder to the feet, especially if you perspire heavily, and wipe antiseptic between the toes.

Personally, I don't recommend men buffing their toenails, but I'll leave the option open. However, some men are now wearing polish. If you choose to do so, just make sure you allow ample time to dry before putting your feet into socks or shoes, as this may mar the polish.

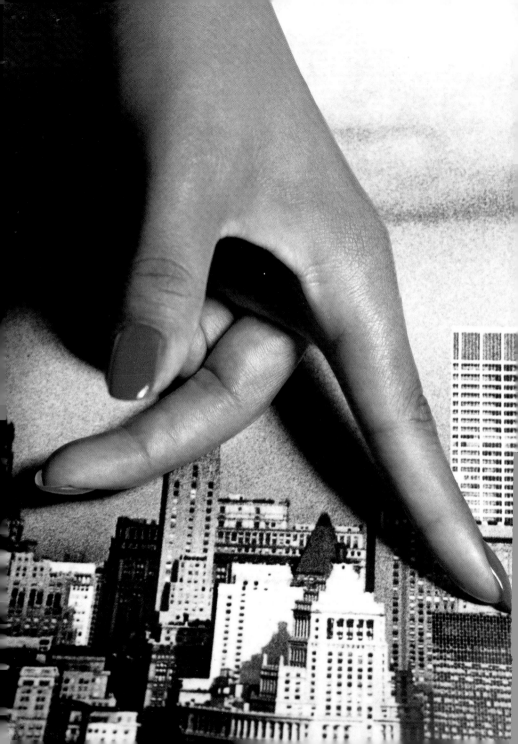

10 Let Your Fingers Do the Walking

(Nail Salons, Cosmetics, Drug, Beauty Supply, and Department Stores)

A great deal has changed in nail care over the years, not the least of which has been the enormous rise in the popularity of nail salons. Once, a manicure or pedicure was something that you'd do at home or in a beauty shop; now you can walk into one of thousands of locations worldwide and get treated to any one of a dozen techniques for the nails only. In many urban centers, salons pop up as frequently as coffee bars. And because of the relative affordability, the opportunity to have well-groomed nails is there for anyone who will take it. But don't view these establishments cavalierly. There are good ones and some not-so-good ones. So there are a few things you should keep in mind before visiting your neighborhood *atelier.* First, look to see how the place is maintained. If it looks disheveled and in disarray, there is a chance this can interfere with a good manicure. Remember, no matter how busy a place is, it should maintain an acceptable level of cleanliness and organization. Second, make sure that the individual manicurist uses the proper hygienic methods with his or her tools. It is very easy and not uncommon to get a nasty nail infection when the tools have not been properly sterilized. If you don't

Classic magenta nails, "out on the town."

see it being done, insist on it! (If you like, you can bring in your own tools and products. This makes some people feel more at ease. But a good manicurist works best with the implements she is most comfortable with. And if she or he is exercising the proper practices, you have nothing to worry about. If however, you have a specific nail color in mind, you might want to bring it along, as choices in some places can be limited.) Third, check for a license (either for the business or the individual manicurist). Many may not have one because it is not a requirement. It's a good idea to check this beforehand, especially if you are going into a salon without a referral to a specific manicurist.

Along with the popularity of the nail salons, there has been a sharp increase in the number of nail products and tools available to the general public. This rise has been attributed to, among other things, the greater affordability of better-quality products, the general accessibility and low cost of professional manicures, the widespread acceptance of better nail grooming habits, and, of all things, the proliferation of the personal computer. But with so many choices comes a dilemma. Where to go to get the best value and the best selection? Usually, it works this way: Beauty supply stores will, more than likely, have the best selection, especially of tools, and at the best prices. They are the favorite haunts of the professionals because you can get things there that you can't find normally

Standing in the doorway of one of my all-time favorite beauty supply stores, Petrucelli's in Queens, New York.

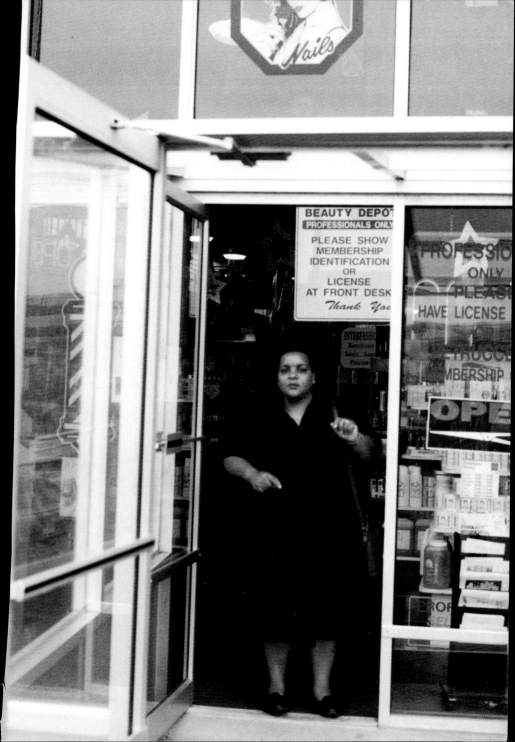

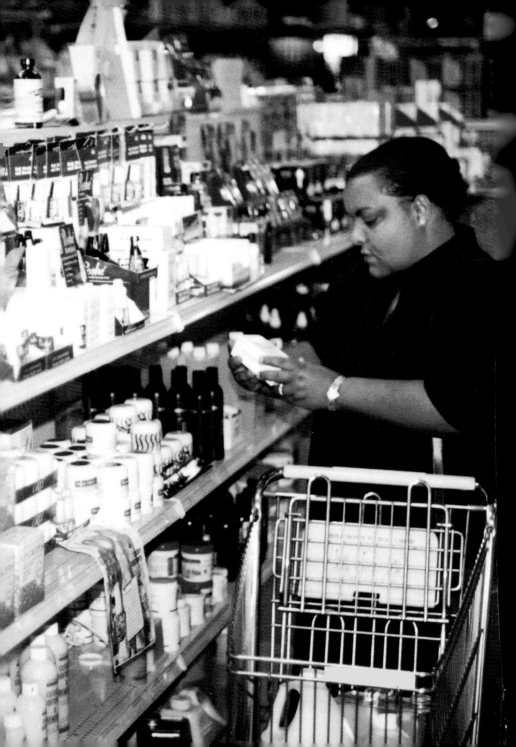

in other places. But there are very few of them around, and they usually cater only to people in the trade. (However, you might be able to find them listed in your phone book under *Beauty Supplies*.) A cosmetics store will, more than likely, have a good selection of tools, but specialize in products in all category levels, from low- to middle- to high-end. A lot of these chains have sprung up in recent years and they are quite popular. Drugstores will usually have some tools and some products but only carry the mass-market brands. They do, however, generally have very good prices. In a department store you won't find many tools, if any, but it may be the only place you'll be able to buy some "designer" nail polishes.

When shopping, avoid buying items on impulse or just because of a good price. If you are not sure you will use them, wait. Remember, polishes and cremes all have a shelf life, so if you don't use them within the next few months after purchase, they may lose their potency. Some tools, though, are used quite frequently, such as emery boards, disk files, and cotton. It might be to your benefit to buy these in bulk, especially because you should not be using worn files on your nails! With implements, such as scissors and clippers, always look to buy the best quality, as they will last much longer. And, always replace a tool that has a worn or dulled cutting edge.

Choose wisely!

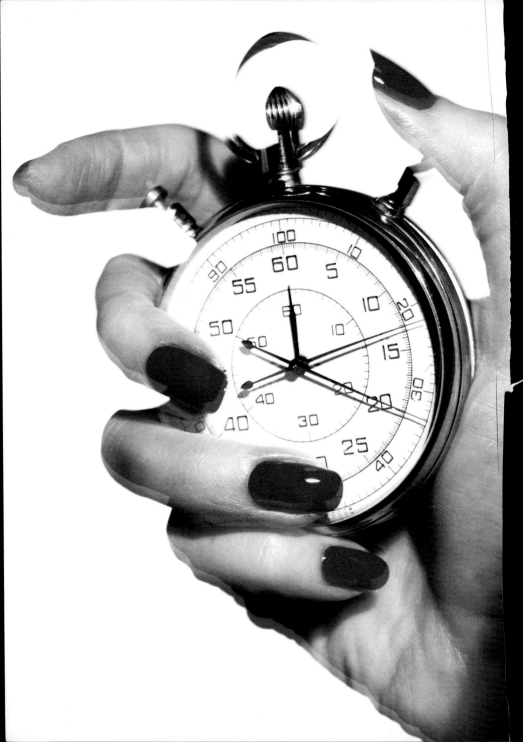

11 Get the Point!
(A Few Important Things to Remember)

The best base coat is a ridge filler. It creates a smooth surface and aids in the application of varnish.

Make sure that nail surfaces are oil- and moisture-free before applying any base coat or varnish to ensure a longer-lasting bond.

Use base coat to prevent colored nail varnishes from yellowing or tinting the nail.

When applying varnish, avoid painting up to the cuticle edge. Varnish can cause the cuticle to become dry and brittle.

Use a cotton swab, dipped in hydrogen peroxide, to whiten and remove stains from the surface of the nail.

The nicotine from smoking increases the chances that your skin and nail polish will yellow.

If you are at the beach, relax by rubbing your heels and palms

Remember always to allow enough time for your polish to dry.

(lightly) in the sand. It acts as a natural abrasive, removing excess skin much like a pumice stone. But don't overdo it!

Push back your cuticles after a bath or shower. (This is when they are at their softest and most pliable. It's also a good way to train them to stay in place.)

Never file your nails when they are wet! (When nails are moist the fibers tend to separate, becoming fragile. Filing them increases the chances of tearing and unneccessary damage.)

Nail buffing is a stimulant for nail growth. However . . .

Excessive buffing of the nails can dry them out. The actual rubbing motion draws the moisture up to the surface. Counter this by moisturizing the nail plate with a buffing creme (or moisturizer).

Buffing is, however, a good alternative for those who are sensitive or allergic to the ingredients in some nail products and varnishes. It gives a great shine that can substitute for polish.

In many states a cosmetological **license** is not required to practice manicuring. Beware!

A quick way to narrow the look of a nail: Apply varnish toward the center, leaving a thin line unvarnished along each side.

Pale-colored nail polishes show less wear and tear, and require less maintenance than dark-colored ones.

Allow some time for coats to dry when applying sheer varnish to prevent uneven application and streaking.

Quick fix: For a night out, dab on a bit of natural oil on dry cuticles for a moist, healthy look.

On special occasions, where your hands are a focus, like weddings, apply a bit of foundation and powder on your hands for a *smoothing* effect.

An orangewood stick dipped in remover (or a polish pen) is a more *controlled* way to clean up misplaced or smeared polish around the nail.

Excessive wetting and drying of the nails and hands (possibly from daily cleaning around the house) can cause splitting and cracking of the nail surface and edges. Always try to wear cotton-lined plastic gloves and moisturize the hands and nails when you are done.

Be patient! Allowing the nails to dry thoroughly will ensure an unblemished, longer-lasting manicure or pedicure.

Use an *acetone-based* polish remover on a real nail and a *non-acetoned-based* one on a synthetic nail.

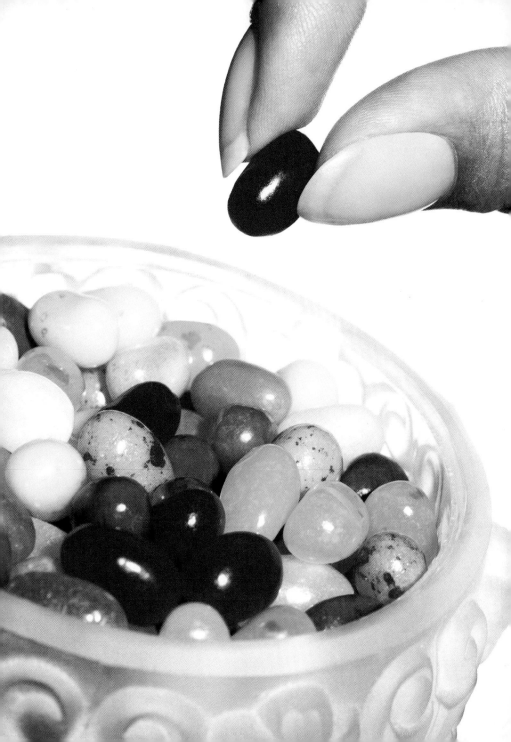

12 At Your Fingertips

(Index and Glossary)

abrasion - a worn area on the surface of the skin, caused by excessive rubbing.

accelerator - a chemical agent that quickens actions, as in a nail dryer.

acetone - a colorless, flammable solvent, used in many polish removers.

acrylic nails - see pages 60–63.

agnail - when the cuticle splits around the nail; hangnail.

alcohol, rubbing - an antiseptic.

antibacterial - prevents the growth of bacteria.

antibiotic - a drug that inhibits the growth of bacteria.

antisepsis - the method by which something is kept sterile.

antiseptic - a chemical agent that can kill bacteria and prevent its growth.

applicator - an instrument used to apply products.

arc - see page 59.

baby basics - see page 39.

base coat - see page 36.

beautician - someone licensed to perform cosmetological functions.

beauty clinic - where cosmetology students can practice skills before moving to a salon.

benzine - a cleaning agent.

bleach - a product that can be used to remove stains from the nail surface.

broken or torn nails - see pages 78–79.

bunion - generally a swelling of the joint of the big toe.

callus - hardened skin on the feet and palms.

carpal - the wrist or wrist area.

certification - completion of course study, as in cosmetology school.

color polish application, basic - see pages 64–65.

cosmetician - a person specializing in cosmetics and their application.

cotton (natural) - see page 29.

cuticle - arc of skin at the base of the finger- and toenails. See page 23.

cuticle care, basic - see pages 48–49.

cuticle oil/creme - see page 36.

cuticle nippers - see page 31.

In nail care today, the choices are yours!

cuticle remover/softener - a liquid substance used in manicures and pedicures to soften cuticle and ease in the removal of excess.

decals, nail - see pages 66–69.

dermatologist - one who treats and understands skin diseases, function, and structure.

digit - another name for finger or toe.

digitus anularis - the ring finger.

digitus demonstrativus - the index finger.

digitus medius - the middle finger.

digitus minimus - the last finger.

disinfectant - a chemical agent used to kill germs and sanitize equipment.

disk file - see page 29.

emery board - see page 28.

enamel - another name for nail polish.

epidermis - the outermost layer of skin.

FDA - the Food and Drug Administration. Federal "watchdog" agency, responsible for overseeing cosmetics and drug companies and their products.

French manicure, modified - see pages 57–59.

fungicide - a product used to kill fungus.

fungus - a parasitic growth. See page 77.

gelatin - a protein extract.

hangnail - a tear in the skin at the side or base of the nail. See page 77.

hydrate - to add moisture.

hydrogen peroxide - a bleaching substance, used also as an antiseptic.

hypoallergenic - less likely to cause allergic reactions.

hyponychium - the thickened layer of skin that lies directly underneath the free edge of the nail.

impermeable - cannot be penetrated.

implement - an instrument or tool.

infectious - likely to cause an infection.

ingrown nail - a nail that grows into the flesh instead of outward, toward the edge.

insoluble - not able or very difficult to be dissolved.

keratin - the fiber protein and principal component present in hair, nails, feathers, and the like.

keratoma - another name for a callus.

ketones - substances used in nail solvents and polishes.

kosmetikos - the Greek word for cosmetics.

lacquer - another name for liquid nail polish.

length, basic nail - see pages 42–45.

lifestyle - see pages 40–41.

lunula - the half-moon, whitish crescent at the back of the nail. See page 23.

macronychia - an abnormally large finger- or toenail.

magnifying glass - see page 32.

manicure - the treatment and care of hands and nails.

manicure, basic - see pages 52–53.

manicure, men's basic - see pages 94–95.

manicurist - a professional who tends to the care and grooming of hands and nails.

mantle, nail - the fold of skin, edged with the cuticle, into which the nail is imbedded.

manus - Latin for hand.

massage, basic - see pages 88–89.

melanonychia - a darkening of the nails.

metacarpus - the bones making up the palm of the hand.

metatarsus - the bones making up the instep of the foot.

micronychia - an abnormally small finger- or toenail.

moons - another name for the lunula.

nail - the horny, keratin-composed protective covering over the ends of the fingers and toes.

nail art - see pages 66–69.

nail bed - the area where the nail rests. See pages 22–23.

nail brush - see page 33.

nail buffer (handheld) - see page 33.

nail buffer (stick version) - see page 30.

nail clippers (two versions) - see page 32.

nail groove - the furrow at the side of the nail, through which it grows. See pages 22–23.

nail matrix - the growing portion of the nail imbedded at the root. See pages 22–23.

nail root - the part of the nail imbedded under the nail fold. See page 22–23.

nail scissors - see page 28.

nail stone (natural) - see page 31.

nail tips - see pages 60–63.

nail wrapping - see page 80.

onych - the Greek word for nail.

onychatrophia - a wasting away of the nail.

onychauxis - enlargement of the nail.

onychia - inflammation of the nail matrix; possibly resulting in the loss of the nail.

onychitis - swelling of the area around the nail.

onychohelcosis - an ulceration of the nail.

onycholysis - a loosening of the nails without loss.

onychomadesis - separation of nail from bed.

onychomycosis - nail fungus disease.

onychopathy - diseases of the nails.

onychophagia - nail biting and the habit of.

onychorrhexis - abnormal brittleness of the nail.

onychosis - any disease or abnormality of the nail.

orangewood stick - see page 30.

pedi - Latin for foot.

pedicure - the care and grooming of the feet and toes. See pages 86–87.

pedicure, men's basic - see pages 94–95.

perionychium - the skin surrounding the nail.

phalanx/phalange - the bones of the fingers and toes.

plantar - relating to the sole of the foot.

podiatrist - a professional who treats the afflictions and diseases of the foot.

polish - common name for liquid product used to coat, protect, and beautify the nails. See page 36.

polish, chipped or smudged - see page 81.

polish dryer - product used to help speed the drying of nail polish.

polish remover - see page 36.

polish remover pad - see page 29.

polish thinner - product to be used when polish has become thickened.

press-on tips - see pages 60–63.

products, general nail - see pages 34–37.

pterygium - forward growth of the cuticle over the surface of the nail.

pumice stones - see page 28.

ring application - see pages 72–73.

sculptured nails - another term used for acrylic nails. See pages 60–63.

shape, basic nail - see pages 44–47.

structure, nail - see pages 22–23.

sheer - see-through.

sole - bottom surface area of the foot.

stearic acid - a white, fatty acid used as a lubricant in powders, cremes, lotions, and soaps.

stone application - see pages 70–71.

synthetic nails - see pages 60–63.

tarsus - the bones of the instep.

titanium dioxide - a white, crystalline powder used in the manufacture of nail polishes to enable coverage.

toe separator - see page 31.

toenail scissors - see page 32.

toluene - a colorless liquid used as a solvent in nail polish.

top coat - see page 36.

topical - limited to the surface of something.

toxic - poisonous.

translucent - clear, enabling light to pass through; similar to sheer.

varnish - another name for nail polish.

viscous - sticky or gummy.

white pencil - see page 29.

zinc - metallic element used in cosmetic powders and ointments.